WALL PILATES FOR SENIORS TO LOSE WEIGHT

Achieve Healthy Weight Loss and Enhance Stability with a 28-Day Program Featuring Step-by-Step Illustrated Pilates Exercises

Carlos McDaniel

Table of Contents

Chapter 1: Introduction to Wall Pilates

In the center of a bustling town, hidden amid cute coffee shops and vivid flower sellers, was a small but dazzling bookshop famed for its one-of-a-kind health and wellness collection. "Wall Pilates for Seniors to Lose Weight" took its place on a bright shelf, eager to improve lives.

The narrative starts with Martha, a vibrant 70-year-old with dazzling eyes and a personality that refuses to age. Martha's enthusiasm for life dwindled after years of struggling with weight gain and arthritis. Walks at the park with her granddaughter got shorter, and her once-loved garden was neglected. The thriving senior community she was a member of appeared to continue on without her.

One clear autumn morning, as golden leaves swirled in the breeze, Martha came upon the book while looking for a new activity to rekindle her passion. She was fascinated by the book, which promised moderate yet efficient weight loss using Wall Pilates. Its cover, featuring a tranquil image of an elderly woman gracefully completing a wall exercise, spoke to Martha like a ray of hope.

Martha turned the pages and learned about the author, Eleanor, a Pilates instructor who specializes in senior fitness. Eleanor had seen firsthand the difficulties elderly faced in maintaining their health and independence. Eleanor was inspired by her grandmother, who used Wall Pilates to restore movement and lose weight, and she committed her life to creating this detailed instruction. It was more than simply a series of activities; it demonstrated the strength of resilience and the notion that age is only a number.

Eleanor's approach was deliberately crafted to appeal to elders, focusing on safety, steady growth, and the joy of exercise. It promised not just weight loss, but also a healthier, more active lifestyle. Each chapter featured a combination of simple instructions, personal experiences, and testimonials from seniors who had altered their lives with Wall Pilates. They spoke of regained mobility, decreased discomfort, greater power, and a sense of success that pervaded their entire lives.

Martha was mesmerized. She recognized herself in these stories: Joan, who could now play with her grandkids without fear of pain; Michael, who had been able to regulate his diabetes and lower his medication; and Linda, who had discovered a new community of friends in her Pilates class. The handbook was more than just a book; it was a gateway to a community of like-minded people seeking health, pleasure, and longevity.

Martha bought the handbook with renewed determination. Within weeks, she noticed a shift. The wall became her buddy and support. She mastered the Wall Roll Down, Standing Leg Lifts, and the Wall Plank. Each day brought fresh strength, and with it came weight loss, not only from her body but also from her soul.

The handbook became Martha's gospel, which she spread not just to her friends but to anybody who would listen. The bookshop struggled to keep up with the demand as more seniors sought the enchantment Martha had discovered within its pages.

"Wall Pilates for Seniors to Lose Weight" was more than a guide; it was a movement, a promise that it is never too late to alter your life. For seniors like Martha, it provided a second opportunity at youth, not by adding years to their lives, but by adding life to their years.

Martha realized the guide was her key to a renewed existence as she looked in the mirror, no longer seeing the weight of age but the lightness of being. It wasn't just about losing weight; it was about entering a world where restrictions vanished and every day carried the possibility of new experiences.

Martha's experience exemplifies the potential of Wall Pilates for anybody at the crossroads of ageing and health, asking if the route to vitality is available. Regardless of the date on your birth certificate, purchasing this book opens the door to a richer, healthier, and more joyous life.

What is Wall Pilates?

Wall Pilates, a variation on classic Pilates, uses a flat vertical surface—the wall—as a tool to improve movements by providing support and resistance. This novel technique is especially effective for seniors wanting to lose weight since it adapts the main concepts of Pilates to the physical limits and demands common to older persons. The wall serves not only as a stabilizer, lowering the risk of injury by assuring perfect alignment and balance, but also as a tool for intensifying workouts by providing leverage and resistance. Because of its dual duty, Wall Pilates is both an excellent and safe workout choice for seniors.

Wall Pilates movements are intended to strengthen the core, enhance flexibility, and boost total muscular tone. For seniors, these advantages are critical, not just for weight reduction but also for improving functional movements required for everyday tasks. The core, being the body's center of power, supports and stabilizes the torso during all activities. Strengthening it can have a considerable influence on one's posture, balance, and stability, hence preventing falls, which are a typical issue for the elderly. Furthermore, the emphasis on regulated, precise movements allow various muscle groups to be engaged at the same time, resulting in more calories expended both during and after a workout.

Unlike other types of exercise that may be too rigorous or high-impact for older people, Wall Pilates provides a low-impact option that is soft on the joints while still demanding enough to achieve weight reduction. The wall is a continuous companion that people may rely on for support, press against for resistance, or utilize to ensure their alignment.

This versatility makes it an excellent workout for seniors of all fitness and mobility levels, allowing everyone to join and profit from the activity.

The breathing methods taught in Wall Pilates are extremely beneficial, particularly for seniors. Deep, regulated breathing not only helps attention and relaxation, but it also increases blood oxygen levels. This enhanced oxygen flow increases energy levels and helps to burn calories more efficiently. Furthermore, the emphasis on breath practice combined with movement fosters a conscious connection to the body, allowing practitioners to become more aware of their physical condition and requirements.

Wall Pilates also promotes independence in seniors by giving them a fitness programmed that they can do in the safety and comfort of their own homes. This accessibility is critical for sticking to a consistent exercise routine, which is necessary for long-term weight loss. The exercises are simply adapted to increase or reduce difficulty, allowing anyone to go at their own speed. This scalability allows seniors to continue to push themselves as their strength and fitness increase, avoiding plateaus in their weight reduction path.

Another important component of Wall Pilates is its community-building potential. While these exercises can be done alone, seniors are urged to participate in groups or supervised workshops. This social connection may be extremely motivating, offering both accountability and support. Sharing experiences, difficulties, and accomplishments with people who share similar goals may help to build a sense of connection and commitment, both of which are vital in sustaining an active lifestyle and losing weight over time.

To summaries, Wall Pilates is a comprehensive approach to weight loss for elders that addresses physical, mental, and social aspects of wellness. Its versatility, safety, and efficacy make it an excellent fitness routine for older individuals who want to reduce weight and improve their general health. Through persistent exercise, elders can enjoy greater mobility, strength, and a higher quality of life, proving that age is only a number, and vitality can be recaptured at any point.

The Science of Pilates for Weight Loss

Pilates, a low-impact workout that focuses on core strength, flexibility, and mindful movement, has been shown to help people lose weight, especially seniors. This strategy, particularly when modified to wall Pilates, provides a safe and effective alternative for older persons to manage their weight since it focuses on muscle strengthening and metabolic improvement. The theory behind Pilates for weight reduction is based on muscle toning and higher metabolic rate. Seniors who do wall Pilates work against gravity and body weight resistance, which aids in the development of lean muscular mass. This is important because muscle tissue consumes more calories than fat tissue, even at rest, therefore the more muscle mass an older adult has, the higher their resting metabolic rate will be.

Wall Pilates, a variation that employs the wall as a source of support and resistance, is especially useful to seniors. It lowers the chance of injury and guarantees that workouts are carried out with optimal alignment and control. This type of Pilates can be very successful at addressing the core, hips, and thighs, which are generally difficult to tone, especially in later age. Wall Pilates requires controlled, precise movements that stimulate many muscle groups at the same time, making it an effective type of exercise for weight management and general strength.

Pilates' mindful element, which emphasizes breathing and focus, is also beneficial for weight reduction. This attention can lead to a greater understanding of hunger and fullness cues, allowing seniors to make healthier food choices and eat more intuitively. Furthermore, the stress-relieving effects of mindful exercise can reduce cortisol levels, which, when raised, can lead to weight gain, particularly in the abdomen. Wall Pilates incorporates mindfulness, which not only benefits physical health but also adds to emotional and mental well-being, which is critical for a comprehensive approach to weight loss.

Another important consideration is adaptability, which makes wall Pilates appropriate for seniors wanting to reduce weight. Exercises may be changed to meet different fitness levels, mobility challenges, or health conditions, allowing everyone to engage safely and efficiently. This versatility means that as elders gain strength and flexibility, the intensity and complexity of the exercises may be increased to keep the body challenged and promote weight reduction.

Integrating wall Pilates into a senior's programmed can provide long-term weight control benefits. Regular practice can improve posture and balance, allowing you to do daily tasks and other types of exercise more effectively. This increase in general activity levels can aid with weight reduction and maintaining a healthy weight over time.

The social component of participation in wall Pilates courses should not be neglected. Joining a class may give elders with inspiration and support, which are essential for sticking to a regular fitness regimen. Being part of a group with similar health and wellness objectives may help to promote consistency and accountability, both of which are essential components of a successful weight reduction journey.

To summaries, the science of Pilates, especially when implemented through wall Pilates for seniors, provides a holistic method to weight loss. It combines physical activity, mindfulness, and social support to address the multidimensional aspect of weight control in older adults. Wall Pilates offers seniors a safe, effective, and comprehensive approach to obtaining and maintaining a healthy weight by emphasizing muscle toning, metabolic rate, mindful eating, stress reduction, adaptability, and community.

Advantages of Wall Pilates for Seniors

Wall Pilates appears as a particularly excellent fitness regimen for seniors, particularly those beginning on a weight reduction journey, due to its unique combination of accessibility, safety, and efficacy. Unlike traditional Pilates, which may need complicated equipment or difficult poses, Wall Pilates uses the wall as a stabilizing aid. This is important for seniors because it minimizes the chance of falls and injuries, which are a significant worry among older persons who participate in physical exercise. The wall serves as both a support and a resistance tool, allowing the practitioner to perform movements with more control and accuracy. This control is essential for targeting specific muscle parts, increasing muscular tone, and assisting in the progressive and healthy reduction of weight.

The versatility of Wall Pilates enables a wide range of exercises to be tailored to specific fitness levels and health problems. The capacity to alter intensity and range of motion is critical for seniors, especially those with chronic diseases like arthritis or osteoporosis. This customisation guarantees that each person may safely conduct activities without worsening pre-existing health conditions. Furthermore, Wall Pilates may be modified to emphasise core strength, balance, and flexibility, all of which are important components in preserving functional independence and lowering the risk of falling, hence aiding weight reduction efforts by allowing for regular and long-term exercise participation.

Wall Pilates also improves posture and alignment, which is very advantageous to seniors. Maintaining appropriate posture becomes more difficult as we become older, due to weakening muscles and diminished flexibility. Wall Pilates routines focus on the core, back, and shoulder muscles, all of which are necessary for proper posture. Improved posture not only reduces back and neck discomfort, but it also improves respiration and digestion, which all contribute to healthier metabolism and weight control.

Wall Pilates has another advantage for seniors: it improves mental wellness. Regular Pilates practice has been demonstrated to alleviate stress, anxiety, and depression, resulting in a more positive attitude on life. This mental health boost is critical for weight reduction because it improves desire and commitment to a regular exercise routine. Pilates' focused breathing and mindfulness improve cognitive performance and emotional well-being, making it a comprehensive approach to health that supports weight reduction objectives from numerous perspectives.

The social component of participation in Wall Pilates courses or groups should not be overlooked. Social connection is critical for seniors' mental health and has a substantial influence on their physical health. Participating in group exercise gives a sense of connection and support, which promotes regular attendance and persistence in weight loss attempts. This social support is frequently a driving force for elders, making exercise a more joyful and anticipated activity.

Furthermore, Wall Pilates helps to enhance balance and flexibility, which are important for everyday activities and general health. The exercises strengthen the muscles that surround the joints, increasing mobility and lowering the risk of damage from falls. This greater physical capability encourages elders to be more active in their everyday lives, which improves weight reduction and overall health.

Finally, Wall Pilates provides a scalable training programmed that may evolve with the practitioner. As strength, balance, and flexibility increase, the exercises can be gradually modified to provide more challenge and advantages. This flexibility not only prevents weight loss plateaus, but it also leads to continued exercise engagement, assuring long-term health advantages and a continuous weight management strategy. Wall Pilates is an appealing alternative for seniors looking to lose weight and enhance their overall health because of its safety, adjustability, and holistic approach.

Safety First: Precautions and Modifications

Starting a journey with Wall Pilates for seniors looking to reduce weight is a potential way to improve their health and energy. To ensure that this trip is both safe and successful, it is necessary to recognize and apply crucial precautions and adaptations customized to older persons' specific requirements. The cornerstone of safety in Wall Pilates is recognizing elders' physical limits and varying abilities, which necessitates a gentle approach that emphasizes slow, controlled movements to avoid strain and damage.

One important precaution is to get a comprehensive health examination before beginning any Wall Pilates practice. Seniors, particularly those with preexisting health concerns such as osteoporosis, arthritis, or heart disease, should obtain medical guidance to verify that Wall Pilates activities are appropriate and safe for them. This preliminary stage assists in identifying any unique dangers and enables for the development of a personalized fitness plan that addresses an individual's health problems, ensuring that the workouts contribute favorably to weight reduction and general well-being without jeopardizing health.

Traditional Pilates movements may require modifications to address the physical restrictions that are typical in seniors. For example, activities that involve reclining on the floor can be modified to the wall to limit the danger of falling and make them more accessible to elders. Such adjustments not only make the exercises more accessible, but they also aid in the maintenance of perfect form, which is critical for maximizing the benefits of Wall Pilates while reducing the risk of injury.

Another important part of safety is the use of adequate warm-up and cool-down exercises. Each session starts with moderate stretching and ends with cool-down exercises, which assist prepare the body for physical activity and aid in recuperation. These techniques are especially beneficial for seniors because they promote blood flow to the muscles, improve flexibility, and reduce muscular stiffness, lowering the risk of injury.

The tempo at which exercises are performed is also an important issue. Seniors are urged to walk slowly and deliberately, concentrating on the quality of movement rather than quantity. This method not only assures the efficiency of each exercise, but also helps seniors to retain balance and stability, which are critical in preventing falls and other accidents.

Wall Pilates for seniors may be substantially safer with proper instruction and supervision from a competent teacher. An experienced senior fitness teacher can provide instant comments on form and technique, change training regimens in real time, and offer encouragement and support. This personalized supervision is crucial in providing a secure and supportive atmosphere in which elders may confidently participate in Wall Pilates.

Finally, listening to one's body and recognizing its signals is critical for preventing overexertion and damage. Seniors should be encouraged to complete exercises at their own speed, taking breaks as required and avoiding any movements that cause pain or discomfort. This self-awareness guarantees that Wall Pilates continues to be a productive and pleasurable element of a senior's journey to weight reduction and increased health, embracing the notion that exercise, at any age, should complement rather than detract from life.

Chapter 2: Getting Started with Wall Pilates

Equipment and Setup

Wall Pilates is a novel method to training for seniors that focuses on gentle, effective exercises that promote weight reduction and general wellness without the use of bulky, expensive equipment. The beauty of Wall Pilates resides in its simplicity and accessibility, allowing anyone to workout using only their own body weight against a wall. This strategy considerably decreases the chance of damage, making it an excellent alternative for seniors wishing to begin their exercise journey safely.

To begin practicing Wall Pilates, you only need a few basic tools, the most crucial of which is a clear, stable wall area. This area should be clear of barriers, with adequate space to move freely in all directions. Adequate space not only assures safety, but also allows for a complete range of motion during exercises, which is essential for effectiveness and maximizing the benefits of the workout. The environment should be well-ventilated and, if feasible, contain natural light to make the workout experience more joyful and stimulating.

Wall Pilates also requires a yoga mat or a non-slip floor mat. Placing this mat directly against the wall cushions the back, hands, and feet, which is very useful for seniors who have sensitive joints. The mat also resists slippage, guaranteeing stability during activities that involve pushing off or leaning against a wall. This simple improvement may considerably increase comfort and safety, making your workout more successful.

Resistance bands are an excellent way to add diversity and challenge to your Wall Pilates exercise. These bands are flexible and inexpensive, and may be used to provide resistance to leg lifts, arm stretches, and other exercises. Seniors may progressively increase the intensity of their workouts by using resistance bands, which promote muscular strength, flexibility, and endurance, all of which are important factors in weight reduction and general physical health.

Another handy item is a tiny, soft workout ball. When positioned between the wall and the lower back or abdomen during specific workouts, the ball can aid with balance and core activation. It also increases the difficulty of the workout, which helps to build the core muscles more efficiently. The ball's suppleness guarantees that it does not create discomfort or strain, making it an ideal tool for boosting Wall Pilates techniques.

A strong chair or ballet barre can be put near the wall for people who are concerned about keeping balance or require additional support. This device provides assistance during standing workouts by offering something to grip for balance. It is especially beneficial for novices or those with balance concerns, since it ensures safety while increasing confidence in doing the exercises. As balance and strength develop, the need for these supports may lessen, allowing for greater flexibility of movement and challenge.

Finally, purchasing in comfortable, breathable gear and supportive, non-slip shoes will significantly improve your Wall Pilates experience. Clothing that allows for an unrestricted range of motion is essential, as is footwear that gives stability and grip, preventing slips and falls. With the proper setup and equipment, seniors may safely enjoy the multiple benefits of Wall Pilates, such as weight loss, increased flexibility, and better overall well-being, making it a highly recommended exercise for individuals seeking to live a healthier, more active lifestyle.

Understanding Your Body's Limitations

When going on a Wall Pilates journey, particularly for seniors looking to lose weight, it is critical to have a profound awareness and respect for one's body's specific limits. This method not only improves the efficacy of the training routine, but it also greatly minimizes the danger of injury. The body's flexibility, muscular strength, bone density, and joint health all naturally vary as people age. These characteristics play an important part in selecting how to approach Wall Pilates, a type of workout that uses the wall as a tool for stability and resistance.

Wall Pilates, by design, is adaptive, making it an excellent choice for seniors. The workouts may be adapted to suit different fitness levels and physical restrictions. However, the key to securely enjoying these benefits is to first analyze one's own physical capabilities. Recognizing and understanding that certain actions may be difficult or even prohibited is not a sign of failure, but rather a step toward a targeted, efficient training regimen. It is about working with the body, not against it, to gradually increase strength and flexibility without putting it under unnecessary pressure.

The notion of progressive growth is important to Wall Pilates. Beginners, particularly seniors looking to lose weight, should begin with the most basic types of exercises to establish a foundation of strength and flexibility. As the body adjusts, more complicated and harder workouts can be added. This gradual approach guarantees that the body is not overburdened, lowering the risk of muscular strains and joint tension, which can be more severe in older persons.

Listening to one's body is essential throughout Wall Pilates workouts. The body communicates via feelings like discomfort or pain, which indicate when to draw back or make an adjustment. Ignoring these cues might result in setbacks, but heeding them fosters a better, more sustainable practice. It's about striking a balance between challenging oneself and being secure and comfortable. This equilibrium is dynamic, necessitating ongoing attention and modifications depending on the body's daily changes.

Integrating good breathing practices is essential for realizing and accepting the body's limitations. Breath control, a key component of Pilates, improves attention and facilitates the execution of moves with precision and safety. It aids in effort management and overstrain prevention, ensuring that activities are carried out correctly and within the body's present capabilities.

The need of a trained teacher or guide cannot be emphasized, particularly for seniors new to Wall Pilates. A professional may provide essential insights into how to tailor workouts to individual needs, provide comments on form and technique, and recommend adjustments to minimize discomfort or damage. They act as a link between an individual's objectives and their current physical state, creating routines that respect the body's limits while challenging it enough to achieve weight reduction and fitness.

Finally, patience is an asset in the context of Wall Pilates for Seniors. The path to weight reduction and increased physical health is slow, particularly when working within the body's limits. Celebrating little triumphs and regular practice will produce outcomes over time, changing limits into strengths. Understanding and obeying the body's cues leads to a rewarding and successful Wall Pilates practice.

Warm-Up and Cool-Down: Essential Practices

Warm-up and cool-down exercises are essential components of any fitness regimen, particularly for seniors who use Wall Pilates to lose weight. These techniques not only prepare the body for the physical demands of the exercises, but they also aid in the winding down process after a session, which is critical for reducing the chance of injury and increasing the overall efficacy of the workout. Wall Pilates' mild nature makes it an excellent choice for seniors, but warming up and cooling down is essential to guarantee safety and optimize benefits.

A warm-up in Wall Pilates is designed to gradually boost heart rate and circulation, therefore relaxing joints and improving blood flow to the muscles. This procedure is essential for seniors because it prepares their bodies for the variety of motions required in Wall Pilates. A thorough warm-up minimizes the likelihood of strains and sprains by increasing muscular elasticity and responsiveness to the workouts. It might involve easy stretching and wall-based movements that mirror the exercises to be done, ensuring that the body is properly prepared for the next session.

Cooling down, on the other hand, involves gradually returning the body to its resting condition. Following a Wall Pilates session, the body should gradually moderate its speed, enabling the heart rate to return to normal and the muscles to rest. This step frequently includes stretches and relaxation methods to assist release any tension that has built up during the workout. This is especially important for seniors since it helps to reduce muscular stiffness and pain, which can make it difficult to stick to a regular exercise schedule.

Breathing methods should be used throughout both the warm-up and cool-down periods. Deep, regulated breathing improves oxygen transport to the muscles while also promoting relaxation and stress reduction. In Wall Pilates, where breath control is an important component, practicing these methods from the start prepares the mind and body for the attention and accuracy necessary for the exercises. Similarly, completing the practice with concentrated breathing helps to reinforce the impression of calm and accomplishment after the workout.

Flexibility is another key advantage of effective warm-up and cool-down practices. Flexibility decreases with age, rendering seniors more prone to injury during physical activity. Warm-up exercises that gently stretch and mobilize the body can help increase flexibility over time, making Wall Pilates routines simpler and more effective. Similarly, stretching can help you calm down and improve your range of motion, which can contribute to long-term mobility.

The influence of these activities goes beyond the physical to the psychological, providing seniors with a systematic strategy to engaging in their exercise program. Starting with a warm-up creates a positive tone for the session, increasing confidence and preparation for exercise. Meanwhile, the cool-down provides an opportunity for reflection and satisfaction, strengthening the commitment to living a healthy lifestyle.

This psychological factor is critical for seniors beginning on a weight loss journey, as it gives them a sense of progress and success.

Finally, incorporating warm-up and cool-down exercises into Wall Pilates for seniors is about more than just physical preparation and recuperation; it is also about providing a comprehensive workout experience. These activities promote a mindful connection between the body and the activity, which improves the overall efficacy of the workout. For seniors trying to lose weight, this holistic approach not only assures safety and minimizes the danger of injury, but also optimizes the advantages of Wall Pilates, making it a sustainable and pleasurable part of their daily routine.

Setting Realistic Goals

Starting a weight reduction and fitness journey with Wall Pilates may be an exciting and transformational experience for seniors, but it all starts with setting realistic objectives. These goals act as a compass, leading seniors through their workout routine while keeping them in line with their skills, health circumstances, and personal desires. Setting realistic objectives is not about restricting oneself; rather, it is about establishing a structured route that recognizes one's present level of physical fitness, possible limits, and the natural improvement that occurs with persistent practice.

Starting with Wall Pilates gives a distinct benefit, particularly for seniors. The wall support offers stability and safety, lowering the danger of harm and increasing the accessibility of workouts. When defining goals in this environment, it's critical to strike a balance between challenge and safety. A reasonable objective could be to learn the fundamentals of Wall Pilates, such as perfect form in wall squats and wall push-ups, before progressing to more complicated activities. This step-by-step method not only boosts confidence, but also provides a progressive growth in strength and flexibility.

In addition to physical goals, it is critical to establish realistic weight loss expectations. Seniors should be aware that while Wall Pilates is excellent for aiding weight reduction and increasing muscular tone, benefits may not manifest immediately. Goals should represent a long-term commitment to consistent practice and patience with the body's rate of improvement. A healthy weight loss rate, customized to one's individual body and health conditions, can promote a more positive and long-term connection with exercise and body image.

Integrating Wall Pilates into one's daily routine necessitates consideration of time and consistency. Realistic goals can include setting up specified times during the week for Pilates practice, beginning with shorter sessions and progressively increasing duration as strength and endurance develop. This helps to create a habit, making exercise a regular component of one's routine rather than a one-time effort. It's about creating a rhythm that works for one's lifestyle, obligations, and energy levels, so that Wall Pilates is both effective and pleasant.

Flexibility in goal planning is another crucial consideration for seniors. Recognizing that growth is not linear allows for changes to workout regimens as needed. This might entail taking a step back if specific activities become too difficult or if health issues develop, and then gradually progressing back to earlier levels. It serves as a subtle reminder that each person's path to greater health via Wall Pilates is unique and individualized.

Accountability is an important factor in attaining goals. For seniors, this might be discussing their objectives with a family member, friend, or a Wall Pilates group, so establishing a support system that supports perseverance and gives inspiration during difficult times. Celebrating milestones, no matter how little, may help people understand the importance of their efforts and the progress they are making toward their goals.

Finally, creating realistic objectives in Wall Pilates for seniors seeking to lose weight entails adopting a comprehensive approach to health and fitness. Regular practice not only provides physical advantages like as increased strength, flexibility, and weight loss, but also mental and emotional well-being. By establishing reasonable, practical objectives, seniors may enjoy the journey of Wall Pilates, experiencing not only the change of their bodies but also the enrichment of their lives, showing that age is simply a number when it comes to adopting a better, more active lifestyle.

Chapter 3: Core Principles of Wall Pilates

Breath Control

Breath control is essential in the practice of Wall Pilates, particularly for seniors beginning on a weight loss journey. This idea goes beyond just inhaling and exhaling, becoming a strong instrument that improves the efficacy of each action, deepens attention, and develops a harmonic connection between mind and body. For seniors, learning breath control in Wall Pilates not only enhances the physical advantages of the exercises, but also helps to reduce stress and improve cardiovascular health.

Wall Pilates' breath control approach is based on conscious, purposeful breathing that is linked with activity. This careful synchronization aids in increasing oxygen intake and ensuring that muscles receive the oxygen-rich blood required for peak performance and recuperation. The technique of focusing on one's breath also helps to center the mind, making for a more aware and engaged workout experience.

To include breath control into Wall Pilates practice, seniors can follow these instructions:

- Start by standing against the wall, feet hip-width apart, and taking a minute to concentrate on your normal breathing rhythm. Examine the rise and fall of your chest and abdomen.
- As you prepare to perform a movement, take a deep breath through your nose, enabling your belly to expand and fill your lungs from the bottom up.
- As you begin the Pilates action, exhale gently through your lips, activating your core muscles and envisioning yourself emptying all of the air from your lungs. This exhale phase is critical for engaging the deep abdominal muscles, which improves stability and power in the exercise.
- Maintain steady, regular breathing when performing exercises that need you to hold a posture against the wall, such as the wall squat. Inhale while holding the position, then exhale as you return to the beginning position.
- Use the rhythm of your breathing to direct your motions. This avoids speeding through the exercises and ensures that each movement is intentional and controlled.
- If you start to lose control of your breathing, halt and take a few deep breaths to reset. It's critical to have a smooth and equal breathing rhythm throughout your practice.

The advantages of adding breath control into Wall Pilates for Seniors are numerous. Physically, it improves oxygenation in the body, which is necessary for calorie burning and so aids to weight reduction. Deep breathing activates the parasympathetic nervous system, which promotes relaxation and stress reduction. Furthermore, breath control enhances pulmonary function, which is especially useful to seniors because respiratory efficiency declines with age.

Furthermore, the focused nature of breath control in Pilates promotes awareness, which can result in a more attentive and joyful workout experience. This conscious participation can increase elders' awareness of their body, helping to minimize harm by ensuring that motions are executed appropriately and safely.

Breath control is more than just a method for Wall Pilates; it is a transforming practice that improves elders' physical, mental, and emotional well-being. Seniors who include conscious breath control into their Wall Pilates program will feel a higher level of involvement with their exercises, leading in more successful weight reduction, enhanced cardiovascular health, and a greater sense of serenity and wellness.

Centering

Centering is an important aspect in the practice of Wall Pilates, especially for seniors beginning on a weight loss journey. This notion emphasizes on physically activating the body's center, or core, as the focal point from which all motions emanate. Centering in Wall Pilates not only improves stability and balance, but it also guarantees that movements are completed efficiently and safely. For seniors, this is especially essential since it helps to reduce the chance of injury while optimizing the advantages of each activity for weight reduction and overall health.

The muscles of the belly, lower back, hips, and buttocks comprise the core, often known as the "powerhouse" in Pilates parlance. Activating these muscles during Wall Pilates exercises improves posture, aligns the spine, and uniformly distributes the body's weight, eliminating undue pressure on any one area of the body. Here are some steps to assist seniors integrate centering into their Wall Pilates routine:

- Begin with Breathing: Before beginning any action, stand against the wall, back straight and feet shoulder-width apart. Take deep, controlled breaths to help you concentrate and engage your core muscles.
- Engage the Core: As you exhale, gently draw your navel towards your spine to activate the core. Imagine you're tightening a belt around your waist. This engagement should be maintained throughout the workout to help stabilize and preserve your spine.

- Pelvic Tilts: With your back against the wall, slightly bend your knees. Tilt your pelvis forward and back to better grasp the movement of your lower spine, and activate your lower ab muscles. This basic dance reinforces the notion of centering.
- Wall Squats for Strength: Place your feet hip-distance apart and focus your core throughout the exercise. Slide down the wall into a squat position before gently returning to standing. This exercise helps to strengthen the core and lower body.
- Wall Push-ups for Upper Body and Core: Face the wall, position your hands slightly wider than shoulder-width apart, and engage your core. Bend your elbows to lower your body toward the wall, then push back to the starting position. This helps to increase upper-body strength while stressing core stability.
- Maintain Alignment: During workouts, always keep your body in proper alignment. Your head should be up, shoulders down, and pelvis in a neutral position, with your core engaged to help support your spine.
- Progress progressively: As your strength and confidence improve, progressively increase the complexity and duration of your workouts while keeping your core as the focal point of all movements.

The advantages of focusing for elders are complex. Seniors can expect to improve their balance by increasing core strength and stability, lowering their chance of falling. Improved core strength also helps to better posture, which reduces back pain and other discomforts caused by improper spinal alignment. Furthermore, core-focused activities can assist tone the stomach region, hence helping weight loss objectives.

Furthermore, the act of focusing has more than just bodily advantages. It promotes a mindful approach to exercise, allowing seniors to focus on the quality of each action while linking their body and mind. This attention can result in a more enjoyable and successful workout experience, fostering a sense of well-being and accomplishment.

Incorporating centering into Wall Pilates practices gives seniors a firm basis on which to safely and efficiently pursue their weight reduction and fitness objectives. Seniors may improve their physical health by concentrating on the core and practicing centering principles, as well as reap the mental and emotional advantages of a balanced and thoughtful approach to exercise.

Concentration

Concentration is a fundamental component in the practice of Wall Pilates, especially for seniors beginning on a weight loss journey and improving their general health. This approach necessitates intense concentration and attention throughout each workout, ensuring that the actions are not only executed safely but also successfully. Concentration in Wall Pilates can help seniors improve the link between mind and body, leading to a better awareness of the purpose and mechanics of each action.

Concentration during Wall Pilates entails three crucial instructions:

- To begin each session, center yourself: Take a few deep breaths, then exhale to remove any exterior problems or distractions. This helps to create a mental space dedicated to your practice.
- picture the muscles you're engaging: Before starting a movement, picture which muscles will be engaged. This mental image directs your attention on the area of work, increasing the efficiency of the exercise.
- Perform movements with intention: In Wall Pilates, every action should be purposeful and controlled, with your mind completely involved in the exercise. This deliberate concentration helps to preserve good form and alignment, lowering the chance of injury.
- Reduce external distractions: Practice in a peaceful, serene environment where you are unlikely to be disturbed. This outward tranquility promotes interior attention.

- Use the wall as a feedback tool: The wall gives continuous tactile feedback during activities. Pay attention to how your body reacts with the wall, and use it to improve your motions and stability.
- Progress slowly: Rushing through exercises might result in a disorganized focus. Move carefully through each exercise, allowing yourself to completely experience the feelings and mechanics of the action.
- Reflect after each session: After each practice, take a few minutes to reflect on the experience. Consider what was difficult, what was nice, and how your focus shifted during the session.

The advantages of focusing concentration in Wall Pilates for Seniors are numerous. For starters, it increases the efficacy of each workout by ensuring that the relevant muscles are engaged and the body is properly positioned, both of which are critical for weight reduction and strength development. Seniors who concentrate can also increase their body awareness, becoming more attentive to the intricacies of their physical well-being and detecting early symptoms of strain or improvement.

Furthermore, concentration has a meditative effect, which reduces tension and promotes mental clarity. This mental advantage is especially beneficial for seniors since it can boost cognitive function and emotional wellness, resulting in a more optimistic attitude on life and their weight reduction journey.

Improved attentiveness during Wall Pilates results in greater balance and coordination. This is critical for seniors not just during their exercise program, but also in daily activities, since it reduces the chance of falls and accidents.

Finally, the exercise of attention goes beyond the Pilates session. The mindfulness and attention developed through practice can benefit other aspects of life, making seniors more present and involved in their interactions and activities. This overall improvement in quality of life, along with the physical advantages of weight reduction and enhanced mobility, demonstrates the significant impact of incorporating the concentration principle into Wall Pilates exercises for seniors.

Control

Control is a fundamental component in the practice of Pilates, particularly Wall Pilates, and it is especially important for seniors beginning on a weight reduction journey. In the context of Wall Pilates, control refers to the careful and focused execution of each movement, which ensures that each exercise is completed with accuracy and stability. This approach is more than simply physical constraint; it also entails a profound connection between the mind and the body, allowing practitioners to engage the proper muscles and maintain perfect alignment throughout their workout.

For seniors, developing control in Wall Pilates can give several advantages. First, it lowers the chance of injury by eliminating abrupt, uncontrolled motions that can strain muscles and joints. Seniors who focus on control may perform each exercise safely, respecting their body's limits and progressively strengthening their strength and flexibility. This focused method also increases body awareness, allowing practitioners to identify and fix any imbalances or flaws in their physique.

Incorporating control into Wall Pilates movements requires many critical instructions:

- Start each exercise with a minute of concentration, mentally preparing your body for the task and synchronizing your breath with your movements.

- Use your core muscles before and during every action. This offers a sturdy basis, supporting your spine and pelvis while increasing the efficiency of the workout.
- Proceed slowly and methodically, rejecting the need to exploit momentum. This guarantees that your muscles, rather than gravity, perform the effort.
- Pay attention to your alignment. Use the wall as a reference to keep your hips, shoulders, and spine in the ideal position.
- Remember to breathe deliberately during the activity. Proper breathing not only helps to retain control but also enhances oxygen flow to the muscles, which improves endurance and performance.
- Finish each action with the same level of focus you started with. Control is more than simply the active component of the exercise; it also includes how you release and transition to the following action.
- Evaluate your technique on a regular basis and make any adjustments. As your strength and flexibility increase, so will your ability to control movements, allowing you to take on more difficult and advanced workouts.

The benefits of mastering control in Wall Pilates are significant, particularly for seniors looking to lose weight. Controlled motions make workouts more effective by targeting specific muscle areas and optimizing calorie burn. This theory also fosters a stronger mind-body connection, which improves mental clarity and lowers stress, all of which are important aspects in weight management. Furthermore, the enhanced accuracy and stability obtained by regulated movements can improve general functional fitness, making daily tasks easier and lowering the chance of falling.

Seniors who prioritize control in their Wall Pilates practice can have a safe, successful, and rewarding journey to weight loss and enhanced well-being. The emphasis on controlled, thoughtful movement not only aids in physical change, but also fosters a more attentive and harmonious relationship with one's body, providing advantages that reach well beyond the Pilates mat.

Precision

Precision is a fundamental aspect in the practice of Wall Pilates, especially for seniors looking to reduce weight and improve their overall physical health. This approach requires painstaking attention to precise form and alignment in each action, ensuring that exercises are not only effective but also safe. For seniors, focusing on accuracy offers two benefits: increasing the efficacy of each activity for weight reduction and muscle toning while lowering the danger of injury.

In the context of Wall Pilates, accuracy entails a great awareness of body alignment against the wall, which serves as a feedback system, assisting practitioners in appropriately aligning their bodies. For seniors starting out on this path, here are some organized guidelines to integrate accuracy into their Wall Pilates routine:

- Begin with Alignment: Before starting any exercise, make sure your back is flat on the wall. This beginning position aids in posture correction and provides a cue for maintaining alignment throughout the activity.
- Activate Core Muscles: Engaging your core is essential for stability and accuracy. Draw your navel towards your spine and keep it there as you execute workouts. This not only strengthens your back but also improves the efficacy of your motions.
- Focus on Slow, Controlled Movements: Rushing through exercises might result in poor form. Execute each exercise gently, focusing on preserving alignment and working the appropriate muscle groups.

- Use Mirrors for Feedback: If feasible, practice in front of a mirror so you can see and correct your form in real time. This visual feedback can help ensure that each posture and movement is executed precisely.
- Breath Control: Add conscious breathing to your practice. Inhale to prepare for activity, then exhale while doing an exercise. Proper breathing improves not just precision, but also focus and fluidity in your practice.
- Limit repeats to Maintain Quality: Rather than striving for a large number of repeats, prioritize the quality of each repetition. It is preferable to execute fewer repetitions with proper form than more repetitions with incorrect form.
- Seek Feedback: Working with a Pilates teacher or a competent partner may give external feedback on your form and technique, allowing you to perfect your practice and ensure you're doing moves precisely.

The advantages of focusing accuracy in Wall Pilates for seniors are numerous. For starters, it guarantees that the workouts focus on the correct muscle areas, which is critical for optimal weight reduction and muscular strength. By concentrating on exact motions, seniors may increase the metabolic burn and toning impact of each exercise, resulting in more substantial health changes.

Furthermore, Pilates' accuracy fosters a stronger connection between mind and body. This focused participation not only improves the quality of each session, but it also promotes overall well-being and body awareness. For seniors, increased bodily awareness can lead to greater balance, lower fall risk, and enhanced functioning in everyday tasks.

Furthermore, focusing on proper form and alignment helps to avoid injuries that might jeopardize fitness objectives and general health. This characteristic of accuracy is especially advantageous to seniors, whose bodies are more prone to strain and damage.

In conclusion, including accuracy into Wall Pilates practice allows seniors to reach their weight reduction goals safely and successfully. Seniors may get the entire range of advantages from Wall Pilates, including physical fitness and weight control, as well as increased mental clarity and quality of life, by moving mindfully and accurately.

Flow

Flow, a basic Pilates principle, emphasizes the significance of fluid, continuous movement throughout the workout. Understanding and implementing flow into exercises may dramatically improve the efficacy of Wall Pilates for seniors, particularly those who are looking to lose weight. Flow ensures that motions are completed gracefully and efficiently, resulting in a smooth transition from one stance to the next. This technique not only helps to sustain momentum but also to engage and strengthen the muscles more efficiently, resulting in increased endurance, flexibility, and, most significantly, calorie burn.

To include flow into Wall Pilates practices for weight reduction, seniors can follow these instructions:

- Begin with a good warm-up that prepares the body for exercise. Gentle stretches and wall rolls can boost blood flow while lowering the chance of injury.
- Practice breathing methods. Inhale deeply through the nose and expel through the mouth to keep a rhythm that promotes movement.
- Begin with easy exercises to lay the groundwork for more complicated sequences. For example, wall squats may be seamlessly transitioned into wall leg lifts, ensuring that the body moves as one unit.
- Concentrate on the quality of movement above the quantity. Each move should be intentional and controlled, starting from

the center and spreading outwards to improve stability and power.

- Visualize the body gliding across space with grace and purpose. This mental image might help you keep a consistent tempo and make seamless transitions between workouts.
- Use the wall as a mobility guide as well as a source of support. For example, moving the hands or feet along the wall can aid in alignment and provide a wider range of motion.
- Finish with a cool-down routine that follows the flow of the workout, gradually lowering the heart rate and stretching all of the key muscle groups used throughout the session.

The advantages of introducing flow into Wall Pilates exercises for seniors are numerous. First, it promotes conscious movement, which can lower the risk of falls and injuries by increasing balance and proprioception. Second, flow adds a cardiovascular component to the Pilates exercise, which is vital for weight loss. The body burns more calories when it moves continually than when it follows a more static training plan.

Furthermore, exercising flow in Wall Pilates enhances movement efficiency, which is especially good for seniors whose energy levels may be lower than before. Seniors may enhance the effect of their training by focusing on seamless transitions and maintaining a consistent pace.

Furthermore, the notion of flow promotes the integration of breath and movement, which increases oxygen absorption and circulation. This increased blood flow increases energy levels and aids in the effective transport of nutrients to muscles, hence promoting recovery and development.

Finally, the rhythmic quality of flowing motions has a relaxing impact on the mind and body, lowering tension and increasing feelings of well-being. This mental clarity and relaxation may be quite motivating for seniors, encouraging them to stick to a regular exercise schedule and helping their weight reduction quest.

Incorporating flow principles into the wall Pilates for elders is a comprehensive approach to fitness, stressing the relationship between mind, body, and breathing. It's not only about reducing weight; it's about developing a sense of harmony and efficiency in movement, which enhances all areas of health.

Chapter 4: Basic Wall Pilates Exercises

Wall Roll Down

The Wall Roll Down is a foundational exercise in Wall Pilates, particularly beneficial for seniors embarking on a weight loss journey. This exercise is designed to stretch and strengthen the spine, improve posture, and activate the core muscles, all of which are crucial for overall mobility and stability. Its simplicity and the support of the wall make it an ideal starting point for seniors, allowing for a gentle yet effective introduction to Pilates practice.

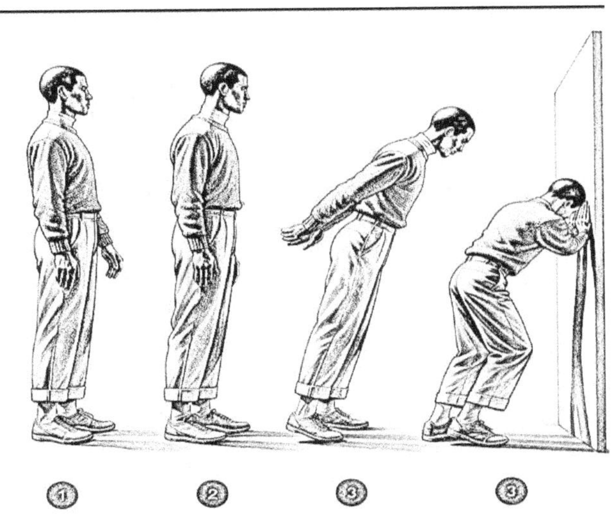

Instructions:

- Start by standing with your back against the wall. Your feet should be hip-width apart and positioned a few inches away from the wall. This stance ensures stability and prepares your body for the movement.

- Allow your arms to hang loosely at your sides, with your shoulders relaxed to avoid any unnecessary tension.

- Inhale deeply, preparing your body for the movement. As you exhale, slowly begin to tuck your chin towards your chest, initiating the rolling down motion from the top of your spine.

- Continue to roll down vertebra by vertebra, peeling your spine off the wall. Keep your abdominals engaged to support your lower back as you descend. Allow your arms to naturally follow the movement, reaching towards the floor.

- Go down as far as comfortably possible without straining. For beginners, it might just be the lower back coming off the wall. With practice, you'll be able to roll down further, increasing the range of motion.

- Pause at the lowest point of your roll down for a moment to deepen the stretch in your spine and hamstrings.

- To return to the starting position, slowly roll back up the wall, pressing each part of your spine against the wall sequentially from your lower back to your neck. Keep your abdominals engaged to support the movement.

- Finish by rolling your shoulders back and down, ensuring you're standing tall with your spine aligned against the wall.

Benefits:

- Improved spinal flexibility: This exercise encourages a gentle stretch along the spine, which can help increase mobility and reduce stiffness, common concerns for many seniors.

- Core strengthening: The act of rolling down and back up requires engagement of the abdominal muscles, which strengthens the core. A strong core is essential for balance, posture, and preventing lower back pain.
- Enhanced posture: Regularly practicing the Wall Roll Down can help correct postural imbalances. It teaches the body to align correctly, reducing the risk of posture-related issues.
- Stress relief: The focused, mindful movement helps release tension in the neck, shoulders, and back, areas where stress commonly accumulates.
- Increased body awareness: Performing this exercise helps seniors become more attuned to their body's movements and alignment, fostering a deeper connection between mind and body.

Incorporating the Wall Roll Down into a regular Wall Pilates routine can significantly contribute to a senior's weight loss and fitness journey. Not only does it provide a gentle yet effective workout, but it also lays the groundwork for more advanced Pilates exercises. By improving core strength, flexibility, and posture, seniors can enjoy a higher quality of life with reduced pain and increased mobility, making the Wall Roll Down an indispensable part of their fitness regimen.

Wall Squat

The Wall Squat is a foundational exercise in Wall Pilates that offers numerous benefits, especially for seniors looking to lose weight and improve their overall physical health. This exercise leverages the stability and support of a wall to ensure safety while effectively targeting the muscles of the lower body, including the quadriceps, hamstrings, glutes, and calves. For seniors, the Wall

Squat is particularly valuable because it strengthens these key muscle groups without placing undue stress on the joints, making it an ideal component of a weight loss and fitness regimen.

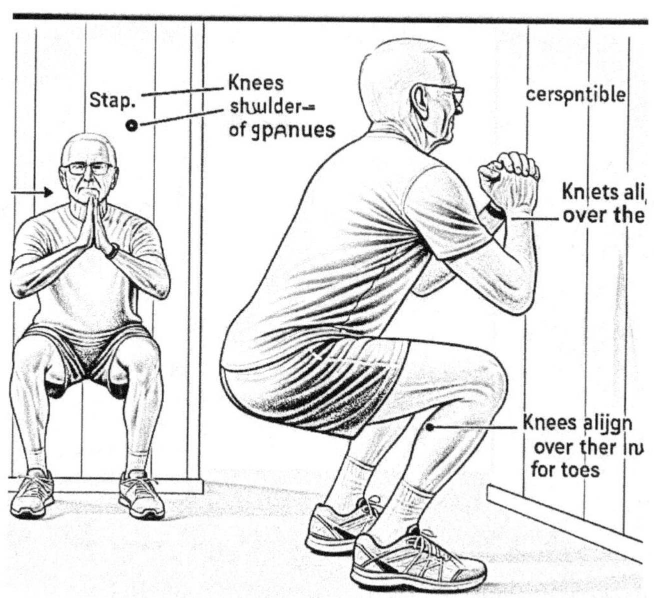

Instructions:

- Start by standing with your back against a flat wall. Your feet should be about hip-width apart and positioned a couple of feet away from the wall, depending on your height.
- Slide down the wall slowly, bending your knees as you go, until your thighs are parallel to the floor. Ensure your knees are directly above your ankles, not extending past your toes, to maintain proper alignment and prevent injury.
- Press your back, especially the lower part, firmly against the wall to engage your core and provide additional support.

- Hold your arms straight out in front of you, parallel to the floor, or place them on your hips, whichever feels more comfortable and helps maintain balance.
- Maintain this position, the squat, for 20 to 30 seconds at the beginning, gradually increasing the duration as your strength improves.
- To return to the starting position, press your feet firmly into the floor and slowly slide back up the wall until you are standing upright.
- Rest for a few moments and repeat the exercise for 2 to 3 sets, depending on your fitness level.

Benefits:

1. Strengthens Lower Body Muscles: The Wall Squat primarily targets the quadriceps, hamstrings, and glutes. Strengthening these muscles is crucial for seniors, as it can improve mobility, balance, and stability, reducing the risk of falls.

2. Improves Joint Health: By aligning the knees and ankles and using the wall for support, the Wall Squat minimizes stress on the joints. This is particularly beneficial for seniors with arthritis or other joint issues.

3. Enhances Core Stability: Although primarily a lower-body exercise, the Wall Squat also engages the core muscles. Maintaining the position against the wall requires abdominal and back muscles to work, thus improving core strength and stability.

4. Aids in Weight Loss: When incorporated into a regular exercise routine, the Wall Squat can contribute to weight loss by building muscle mass. Increased

muscle mass boosts metabolism, which helps the body burn more calories even at rest.

5. Increases Flexibility and Range of Motion: Regularly performing Wall Squats can enhance flexibility in the hips and lower back, contributing to a greater range of motion. This can make daily activities easier and more enjoyable.

6. Safe and Accessible: The Wall Squat is a safe exercise for seniors because the wall provides support, reducing the risk of losing balance and falling. It's an accessible exercise that can be performed at home, requiring no special equipment.

7. Customizable: The exercise can be modified to suit different fitness levels. For beginners or those with knee issues, not going as low into the squat can reduce strain. As strength and flexibility improve, the depth of the squat and the duration of the hold can be increased.

Incorporating Wall Squats into a regular Wall Pilates routine offers a simple yet effective way for seniors to enhance their physical health, contribute to weight loss, and improve their quality of life. As with any exercise program, it's important to consult with a healthcare provider before starting, especially for individuals with pre-existing health conditions.

Leg Circles Against the Wall

Leg Circles Against the Wall are a fundamental exercise in Wall Pilates, particularly beneficial for seniors aiming to lose weight and enhance their overall physical health. This exercise targets the core, hips, and leg muscles, promoting strength, flexibility, and stability. For seniors, incorporating Leg

Circles into their Wall Pilates routine can offer numerous benefits, including improved circulation, enhanced mobility, and a gentle yet effective way to engage and tone the body.

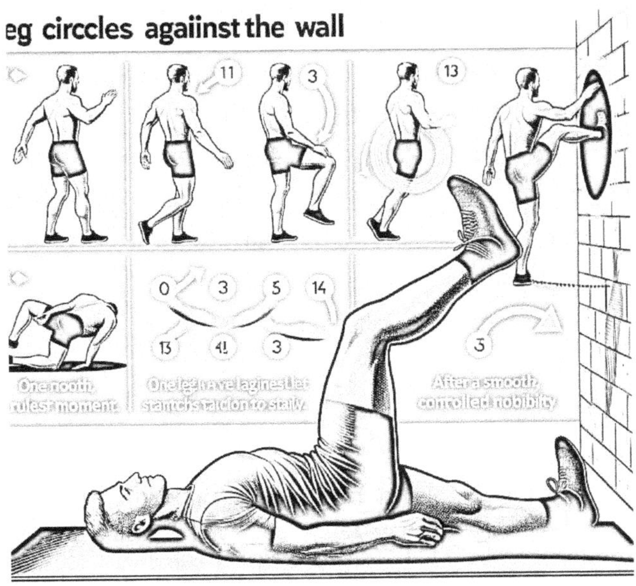

Instructions:

- Start by lying on your back on a comfortable mat, with your buttocks close to and facing a wall. Ensure that your environment is safe and free of obstacles.
- Extend your legs upward, pressing them gently against the wall. Your body and legs should form a 90-degree angle. Place your arms flat on the ground beside you, palms down, to support your body.

- Engage your core by gently pulling your navel towards your spine. This engagement is crucial for stability and ensures that your lower back remains pressed lightly against the floor.
- Begin with one leg (start with the right leg if you're right-handed, or the left leg if you're left-handed), keeping it straight. Lower the other leg down the wall until it's hovering above the ground or at a height that feels comfortable and manageable for you.
- Slowly circle the raised leg in a controlled manner. You can start with small circles, gradually increasing the size as your flexibility and confidence improve. Ensure that the movement is initiated from the hip joint, not just the foot.
- Complete a set of circles in one direction, then reverse the direction for the same leg. A good starting point is 5-10 circles in each direction, gradually increasing as you become more comfortable with the exercise.
- Repeat the process with the opposite leg, ensuring equal attention and effort on both sides.

Benefits:

The Leg Circles Against the Wall exercise offers a range of benefits, especially suited to the needs and capabilities of seniors:

1. Strengthens Core Muscles: The engagement of the core throughout this exercise helps to strengthen the abdominal muscles, which are essential for balance, posture, and everyday movements.
2. Improves Hip Mobility: The circular motion helps to lubricate the hip joints, increasing their range of motion and reducing stiffness or discomfort, which is particularly beneficial for seniors.

3. Enhances Leg Muscle Tone: This exercise targets not just the core but also the thighs and calves, promoting lean muscle development which is key in boosting metabolism and aiding weight loss.

4. Increases Circulation: The movement of the legs against gravity can help improve blood circulation, which is important for overall health and can aid in the prevention of swelling and varicose veins.

5. Promotes Flexibility: Regular practice of Leg Circles can increase flexibility in the hips and legs, contributing to a greater ease of movement in daily activities.

6. Supports Balance and Stability: By strengthening the core and leg muscles, seniors can enjoy better balance and stability, reducing the risk of falls.

7. Low Impact: This exercise is gentle on the joints, making it an ideal choice for seniors or individuals with joint issues, as it offers a safe way to exercise without putting undue stress on the body.

Incorporating Leg Circles Against the Wall into a regular Wall Pilates routine can be a stepping stone towards achieving weight loss goals, improving physical health, and enhancing the quality of life for seniors. It's a testament to the adaptability of Pilates exercises to meet the needs of aging bodies, providing a path to maintaining fitness and independence with age.

Wall Push-Ups

Wall push-ups are a fundamental exercise within the Wall Pilates repertoire, especially designed for seniors embarking on a journey to lose weight and enhance overall fitness. This exercise adapts the traditional floor push-up, making it more accessible and less intimidating for those with limited mobility or strength. Wall push-ups target the upper body, particularly the chest, shoulders, and triceps, while also engaging the core muscles, providing a comprehensive workout that builds strength without the need for equipment.

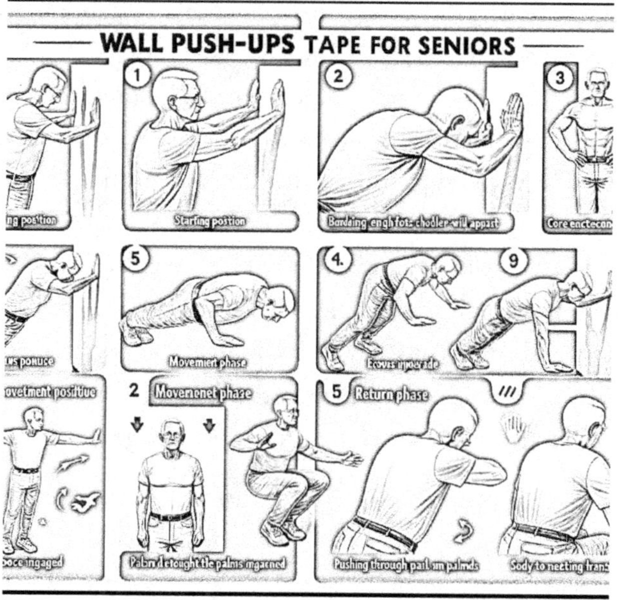

Instructions:

- Stand facing a wall, approximately an arm's length away, with feet shoulder-width apart.

- Place your palms flat against the wall at shoulder height and shoulder-width apart.
- Engage your core and glutes to stabilize your body, ensuring a straight line from your head to your heels.
- Inhale as you slowly bend your elbows, bringing your chest towards the wall in a controlled manner. Keep your elbows pointing downwards rather than flaring out to the sides.
- Pause briefly when your face is close to the wall, ensuring your body remains straight and engaged.
- Exhale as you push through your palms to extend your arms, returning to the starting position.
- Repeat for the desired number of repetitions, starting with a manageable set and gradually increasing as your strength improves.

Benefits:

1. Improved Upper Body Strength: Regularly performing wall push-ups strengthens the chest, shoulders, and arms, which can enhance the ability to perform daily activities such as lifting groceries or reaching for items on high shelves.

2. Increased Core Stability: This exercise requires engagement of the abdominal muscles, which helps to improve posture, balance, and stability, reducing the risk of falls.

3. Enhanced Joint Health: Wall push-ups are low-impact and place less strain on the wrists, elbows, and shoulders compared to traditional push-ups, making them ideal for seniors with joint concerns.

4. Weight Management: As part of a Wall Pilates routine, wall push-ups help in burning calories and building muscle mass, contributing to weight loss and the prevention of obesity-related health issues.

5. Accessibility: The simplicity of wall push-ups allows them to be performed anywhere there is a wall, making it easier for seniors to incorporate regular physical activity into their daily routine without the need for special equipment or a gym membership.

6. Adaptability: The intensity of the exercise can be easily adjusted by changing the distance of the feet from the wall, allowing for a personalized workout that progresses with the individual's fitness level.

7. Mental Health Benefits: Engaging in physical activity like Wall Pilates and wall push-ups can also improve mental health by reducing symptoms of depression and anxiety, boosting mood, and enhancing overall well-being.

Incorporating wall push-ups into a regular Wall Pilates routine offers seniors a safe and effective way to build strength, improve functional abilities, and contribute to a weight loss plan. As with any exercise program, it's important for seniors to consult with a healthcare provider before beginning, to ensure the exercises selected are appropriate for their individual health status and fitness goals.

Standing Leg Lifts

Standing Leg Lifts are a foundational exercise in Wall Pilates that offer a range of benefits, especially for seniors looking to lose weight and improve their overall physical fitness. This exercise targets multiple areas of the body, including the core, hips, and legs, making it a versatile addition to a senior's exercise regimen. Despite its simplicity, the effectiveness of Standing Leg Lifts in building strength, enhancing stability, and promoting flexibility cannot be overstated.

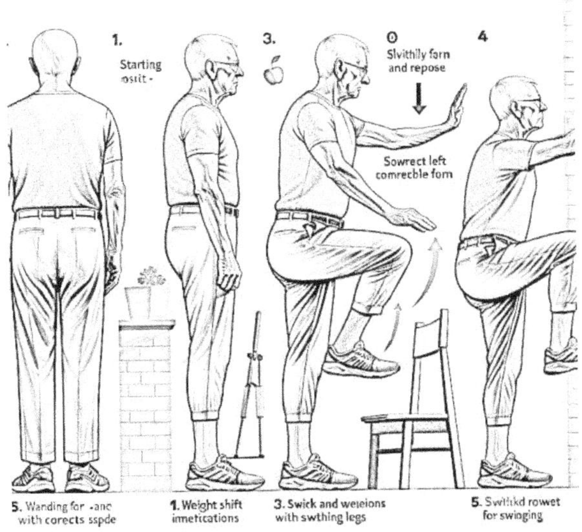

Instructions:

- Begin by standing with your back against a wall. Ensure that your spine is straight, with your head, shoulders, and back touching the wall. This posture helps in engaging the core muscles from the start.

- Place your feet shoulder-width apart for stability. Your arms can rest by your sides, with your palms facing inwards or lightly pressed against the wall for additional support.
- Shift your weight slightly onto your right foot while keeping both feet flat on the ground. This shift prepares your body for the lift.
- Slowly raise your left leg to the side, keeping it straight. Lift it as high as comfortably possible without compromising your form or balance. The goal is not height but maintaining a controlled, stable lift.
- Hold the lifted position for a moment, then slowly lower your leg back to the starting position. This controlled movement is crucial for maximizing the exercise's benefits.
- Repeat the exercise for a set number of repetitions before switching legs.
- Throughout the exercise, keep your movements smooth and controlled. Avoid jerky motions or swinging your leg, as these can lead to strain.

The benefits of Standing Leg Lifts for seniors, especially those focused on weight loss, are multifaceted. Firstly, this exercise aids in toning and strengthening the muscles of the lower body, including the glutes, thighs, and calves. Stronger muscles not only improve mobility and balance but also increase metabolic rate, which is beneficial for weight management.

Additionally, Standing Leg Lifts engage the core muscles, promoting better posture and reducing the risk of lower back pain—a common concern among seniors. The stabilizing effect of these lifts enhances balance, decreasing the likelihood of falls.

Another significant benefit is the improvement of hip flexibility and joint health. By moving the legs in a controlled manner, seniors can maintain or even increase their range of motion in the hips, which is essential for daily activities and overall quality of life.

For seniors embarking on a weight loss journey, incorporating Standing Leg Lifts into their Wall Pilates routine offers a low-impact, safe exercise option that yields significant physical benefits. Regular practice can lead to improved muscle tone, enhanced stability and balance, and a more active metabolism, all of which contribute to healthy weight loss and a more vibrant, active lifestyle.

Moreover, the simplicity and accessibility of Standing Leg Lifts make them an ideal starting point for seniors new to exercise. They require no special equipment and can be modified to suit individual fitness levels, ensuring that everyone can participate and benefit from this effective exercise.

Chapter 5: Intermediate Wall Pilates Exercises

Wall Plank

The Wall Plank, as part of intermediate Wall Pilates exercises, is a transformative activity for seniors aiming to lose weight and strengthen their core, without the strain that traditional floor planks might impose. This exercise leverages the stability of the wall to provide a safer alternative, ensuring that seniors can engage in effective strength training while minimizing the risk of injury.

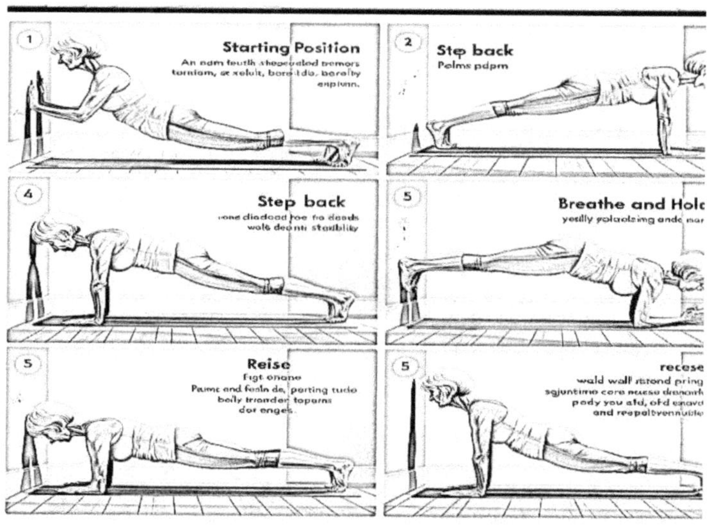

Instructions:

- Begin by facing the wall, standing arm's length away. Place your palms flat against the wall at shoulder height and shoulder-width apart.
- Step back with both feet until your body is leaning forward into a diagonal plank position, with your feet firmly planted on the ground. Ensure your body forms a straight line from your head to your heels, engaging your core to keep your hips from sagging.
- Hold this position, pressing your palms into the wall and keeping your shoulders down and back, away from your ears. Your gaze should be neutral, looking at a spot on the wall to maintain neck alignment.
- Breathe deeply and hold the plank for a duration that feels challenging yet achievable, starting with 20-30 seconds and gradually increasing as your strength improves.
- To release, gently walk your feet towards the wall and stand upright, taking a moment to relax before repeating the exercise.

The benefits of incorporating the Wall Plank into a senior's Wall Pilates routine are multifaceted. Primarily, it strengthens the core muscles, including the abdominals, back, and sides, which are crucial for improving balance and stability—key components in preventing falls and maintaining independence. Additionally, this exercise engages the shoulders, arms, and legs, providing a comprehensive strength training that supports weight loss by increasing muscle mass and boosting metabolism.

Beyond its physical advantages, the Wall Plank promotes concentration and mental endurance. Holding the position requires focus and breathing control, which can enhance mental clarity and reduce stress. For seniors, this aspect of Wall Plank can be particularly beneficial, offering a moment of mindfulness and a sense of achievement as they progress in their ability to hold the plank for longer periods.

This exercise also offers versatility. Seniors can adjust the difficulty level by altering their distance from the wall—standing closer for a less intense workout or further away to increase the challenge. Such adaptability ensures that the Wall Plank remains suitable for a wide range of fitness levels, from those just starting their weight loss journey to more experienced individuals seeking to maintain their strength and mobility.

Incorporating the Wall Plank into a regular Wall Pilates routine can significantly contribute to a senior's weight loss goals, offering a safe, effective method for building strength and endurance. It exemplifies how Pilates, adapted to the needs and abilities of seniors through modifications like the use of a wall for support, can offer a comprehensive approach to health and wellness, emphasizing not only physical fitness but also mental resilience and overall quality of life.

Side Wall Lifts

Side Wall Lifts are a pivotal component of the intermediate Wall Pilates exercises designed specifically for seniors aiming to lose weight and enhance their physical health. This exercise, while seemingly simple, targets and strengthens the obliques, improves balance, and enhances coordination, making it an essential practice for seniors. By leveraging the stability and support of a wall, seniors can safely execute this exercise, minimizing the risk of falls and ensuring a focus on proper form.

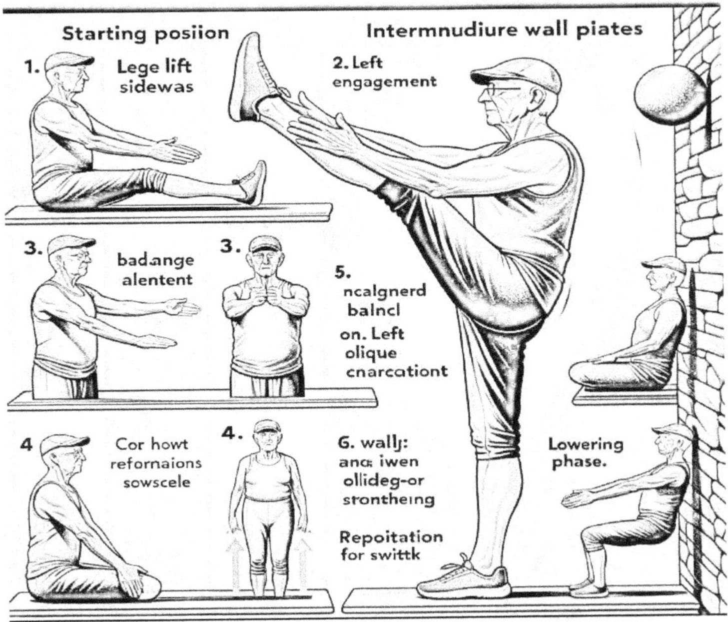

instructions:

- Stand with your right side facing the wall, ensuring your feet are hip-width apart for stability.

- Place your right hand on the wall at shoulder height for support. Extend your left arm down the side of your body.
- Engage your core muscles to maintain balance and alignment throughout the exercise.
- Slowly lift your left leg sideways, keeping it straight, as high as comfortably possible without compromising your posture. Your right arm can apply gentle pressure on the wall for balance.
- Hold the lifted position for a moment, focusing on the contraction in your left oblique muscles.
- Gently lower your left leg back to the starting position in a controlled manner.
- Repeat the lift for a set number of repetitions before switching sides to ensure balanced strengthening on both sides of the body.

Incorporating Side Wall Lifts into a Wall Pilates routine offers numerous benefits for seniors, particularly those focused on weight loss and improving physical strength. Firstly, this exercise directly targets the oblique muscles, which are crucial for core stability and strength. A stronger core not only aids in performing daily activities with ease but also improves posture and reduces the risk of back pain.

Moreover, Side Wall Lifts help in enhancing balance and coordination. For seniors, maintaining balance is vital to prevent falls, which can lead to significant injuries. As balance improves, seniors can feel more confident in their movements, both during exercise and in daily life.

This exercise also contributes to weight loss efforts. By building lean muscle in the core and improving overall strength, seniors can experience an increase in their resting metabolic rate. Muscle tissue burns more calories at rest compared to fat tissue, meaning that an increase in muscle mass can help seniors burn more calories throughout the day, aiding in weight loss.

Additionally, Side Wall Lifts are low-impact and joint-friendly, making them suitable for seniors with varying fitness levels and those with joint concerns. The support of the wall ensures that the exercise can be performed safely, reducing the strain on the knees, hips, and back.

To maximize the benefits of Side Wall Lifts and support weight loss goals, seniors should aim to incorporate this exercise into their routine 2-3 times a week, along with other Wall Pilates exercises. It's also important to combine this physical activity with a balanced diet and adequate hydration for optimal health and weight management.

In conclusion, Side Wall Lifts offer a safe, effective way for seniors to strengthen their core, improve balance, and aid in weight loss. By following the instructions carefully and incorporating this exercise into a regular Wall Pilates routine, seniors can enjoy the myriad benefits it offers, contributing to a healthier, more active lifestyle.

Wall Bridging

Wall Bridging, as an intermediate exercise in Wall Pilates, offers a unique blend of benefits, especially for seniors focusing on weight loss and improved physical fitness. This exercise targets the core, glutes, hamstrings, and lower back, providing a comprehensive workout that enhances stability, strength, and flexibility. Unlike traditional floor bridging, Wall Bridging incorporates the stability of a wall to offer additional support, making it an ideal exercise for seniors who may require more balance and security during their workout routines.

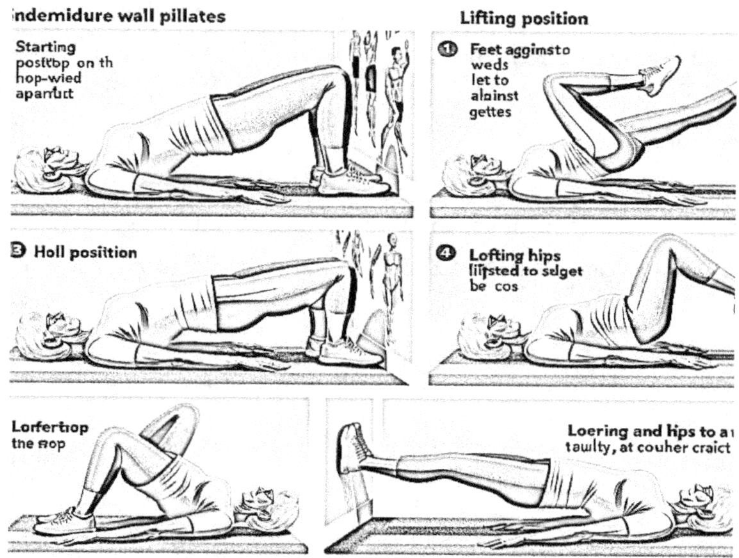

Instructions:

- Begin by lying on your back with your feet flat on the floor, hip-width apart. Your legs should be bent, and your arms rested by your sides.

- Move your feet closer to the wall and lift them so that your soles are flat against the wall, knees bent at a 90-degree angle.
- Pressing your feet into the wall, engage your core and glutes to lift your hips off the floor, aiming to create a straight line from your shoulders to your knees.
- Hold this position for a few seconds, focusing on maintaining a tight core to support your lower back.
- Slowly lower your hips back to the starting position without letting them touch the floor, and then lift again.
- Perform this movement for a recommended set of 10 to 15 repetitions, ensuring smooth, controlled motions throughout.

The benefits of Wall Bridging for seniors, particularly those aiming to lose weight, are multifaceted. Firstly, this exercise helps to strengthen the core muscles, which is essential for improving balance and stability, reducing the risk of falls. Strengthening the core also aids in performing daily activities with more ease and less strain on the body.

Additionally, Wall Bridging activates the glutes and hamstrings, muscles that are critical for posture and lower body strength. By engaging these large muscle groups, seniors can increase their metabolism, which in turn aids in weight loss and the management of body fat. This increased muscle activity contributes to a higher resting metabolic rate, meaning the body burns more calories even when at rest.

Wall Bridging also offers therapeutic benefits, particularly for those with lower back pain. By strengthening the lower back and improving the flexibility of the spine, seniors can experience relief from chronic pain, enhancing their overall quality of life. Moreover, the controlled movement and focus required during

Wall Bridging promote mindfulness and concentration, contributing to mental well-being.

For seniors looking to enhance their Wall Pilates routine for weight loss and improved fitness, incorporating Wall Bridging can provide a gentle yet effective way to build strength, improve balance, and increase flexibility. As with any exercise program, it's important to consult with a healthcare provider or a certified Pilates instructor to ensure the exercises are performed safely and effectively, tailored to one's individual health status and fitness level.

Wall Clock

The "Wall Clock" exercise is a distinctive intermediate-level movement within the Wall Pilates repertoire, specifically designed for seniors focusing on weight loss and overall body conditioning. This exercise, rooted in the principles of Pilates, emphasizes controlled movements, balance, and the strengthening of various muscle groups. Unlike traditional Pilates exercises performed on the mat or with equipment, the "Wall Clock" utilizes the wall as a stabilizing tool, making it particularly suitable for seniors who may require additional support to maintain balance and posture.

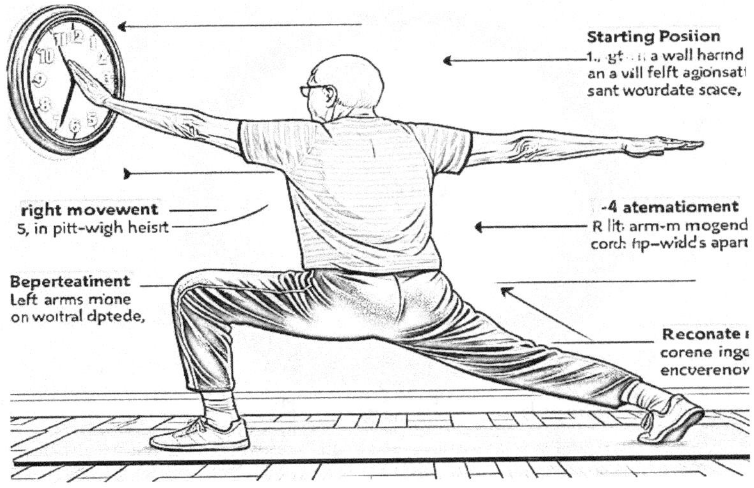

The premise of the "Wall Clock" exercise involves standing at arm's length from the wall, facing away, and using the arms to mimic the hands of a clock. This movement pattern engages the core, shoulders, and back, while also improving flexibility and balance. To perform the "Wall Clock" effectively, follow these instructions:

- Begin by standing with your feet hip-width apart, approximately an arm's length away from the wall. Ensure your feet are firmly planted and your spine is in a neutral position.
- Extend your arms behind you and place your palms flat against the wall at waist height, fingers pointing upwards.
- Engaging your core, slowly move your right hand upwards as if tracing the numbers on a clock face, reaching as high as comfortably possible without straining your shoulder.
- Simultaneously, slide your left hand down towards the lower numbers of the clock face, maintaining a smooth, controlled movement.
- Pause briefly when your arms are fully extended in opposite directions, then slowly return to the starting position at waist height.
- Repeat the movement with your left arm moving upwards and your right arm moving downwards.
- Perform this sequence for a set number of repetitions, typically 8-10 on each side, focusing on the fluidity and precision of the movement.

The benefits of incorporating the "Wall Clock" into a senior's Wall Pilates routine are manifold. Primarily, this exercise targets the core muscles, which are crucial for balance and stability, reducing the risk of falls. The rotational movement also improves shoulder mobility and flexibility, which can be particularly beneficial for seniors experiencing stiffness or limited range of motion in their upper body. Additionally, the "Wall Clock" helps to strengthen the back muscles, supporting proper posture and alleviating back pain, a common concern among the senior population.

Furthermore, the "Wall Clock" contributes to weight loss efforts by engaging multiple muscle groups simultaneously, increasing the body's metabolic rate during and after the exercise. This elevation in metabolism aids in more efficient calorie burn, which, when combined with a balanced diet and regular Pilates practice, can lead to healthy weight loss.

In summary, the "Wall Clock" exercise offers a comprehensive workout that addresses several key areas important for seniors' health and well-being. By improving balance, flexibility, and muscle strength, and contributing to weight loss, this intermediate Wall Pilates exercise is a valuable addition to any senior's fitness regimen. Its unique use of the wall as a supportive tool also makes it accessible to those who might find other forms of exercise challenging, ensuring that seniors can safely and effectively work towards their fitness goals.

Wall Scissors

The Wall Scissors exercise is an intermediate-level Wall Pilates movement that offers a unique blend of balance, core stability, and lower body strength. Specifically designed for seniors aiming to lose weight and enhance their physical fitness, this exercise incorporates the stability of the wall to ensure safety while challenging the body in a gentle yet effective manner. Here's a deeper look into the Wall Scissors, including step-by-step instructions and the benefits associated with this exercise.

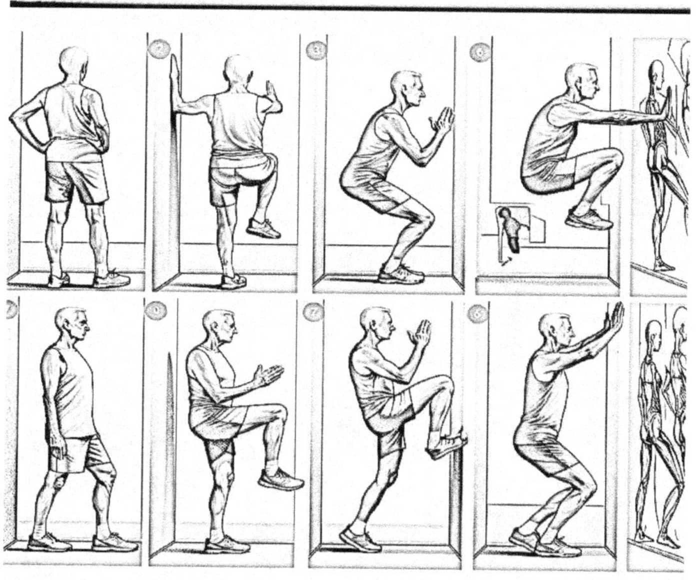

Instructions:

- Start by standing with your back against a wall, ensuring that your spine is straight and your feet are shoulder-width apart. This initial position helps in maintaining proper posture throughout the exercise.

- Walk your feet out slightly from the wall while keeping your back flat against the wall's surface. Bend your knees slightly to get into a shallow squat, engaging your core muscles for added stability.
- Carefully lift your right leg and extend it forward, keeping the leg straight. The toes of your extended foot should be pointed, and the weight of your body should be supported by your left leg and the wall.
- Slowly lower your right leg and simultaneously lift your left leg, mimicking a scissor motion. The movement should be controlled and deliberate, focusing on the stability of your core and the strength of your leg muscles.
- Continue alternating legs in a smooth, scissor-like motion for a set number of repetitions or a set time period, ensuring that your back remains flat against the wall throughout the exercise.
- To increase the challenge as you progress, you can lower into a deeper squat or increase the speed of the leg movements, always paying attention to maintaining form and balance.

Benefits:

1. Improved Core Stability: The Wall Scissors exercise engages the abdominal and lower back muscles, enhancing core stability. A strong core is essential for overall movement efficiency and injury prevention, making daily activities easier and safer for seniors.
2. Enhanced Lower Body Strength: This exercise targets the quadriceps, hamstrings, and glutes, helping to build strength in the lower body. Stronger leg muscles contribute to better balance and mobility, which are crucial for seniors in preventing falls and maintaining independence.
3. Increased Flexibility and Range of Motion: The leg lifting action helps to stretch the leg muscles, promoting flexibility and increasing

the range of motion. This is particularly beneficial for seniors, as flexibility tends to decrease with age.

4. Weight Loss and Improved Metabolism: By engaging multiple muscle groups simultaneously, the Wall Scissors exercise helps to burn calories and can contribute to weight loss efforts. Regular participation in such exercises can also boost metabolism, further aiding in weight management.

5. Low Impact on Joints: The support of the wall and the controlled motion of the legs ensure that this exercise is low impact, making it suitable for seniors with joint concerns or those new to exercise. It offers a way to strengthen and tone without the risk of injury associated with high-impact activities.

Incorporating Wall Scissors into a regular Wall Pilates routine provides a multifaceted approach to fitness for seniors. Not only does it help in weight loss by engaging major muscle groups and boosting metabolism, but it also improves functional fitness, enhancing the ability to perform everyday activities with ease and confidence. As with any exercise program, seniors should consult with a healthcare provider before starting Wall Pilates, ensuring that it's a safe and appropriate option for their individual health needs.

Chapter 6: Advanced Wall Pilates Exercises

Wall Jackknife

The Wall Jackknife is an advanced Wall Pilates exercise that stands out for its effectiveness in engaging the core, improving flexibility, and enhancing overall body strength, making it an excellent choice for seniors aiming to lose weight and elevate their fitness levels. This exercise, while advanced, can be modified to suit the needs and abilities of seniors, ensuring they can safely reap its benefits without compromising on safety.

The Wall Jackknife primarily targets the abdominal muscles, but its execution also recruits the shoulders, back, and leg muscles, providing a comprehensive workout. The movement involves a combination of balance, strength, and control, as it requires the practitioner to lift their legs against the wall while maintaining a controlled motion. For seniors, this exercise not only aids in strengthening the core and improving posture but also contributes to the enhancement of balance and stability, which are crucial for preventing falls and improving functional daily movements.

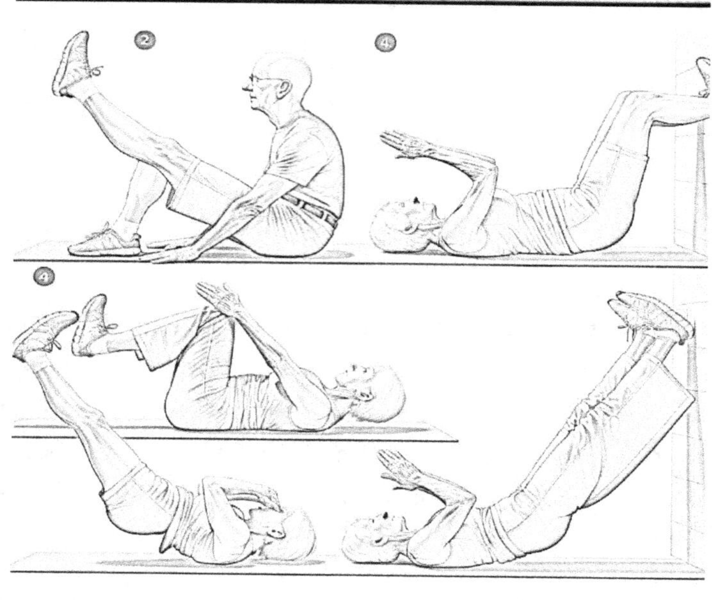

Instructions for performing the Wall Jackknife with modifications for seniors include:

- Begin by lying on your back a few feet away from the wall, with your legs extended straight towards it. Adjust your distance from the wall based on your flexibility and strength.
- Place your hands flat on the ground beside you for support, or if you need extra stability, extend your arms above your head on the floor.
- Slowly walk your feet up the wall until your body forms an L-shape, with your hips aligned directly under your feet. Keep your core engaged and your back straight.
- Inhale deeply, and as you exhale, slowly lift your hips off the ground, pressing your feet into the wall for leverage. Your body should move towards a V-shape, with your legs and torso forming the two lines of the "V."

- Hold this position for a few seconds, focusing on tightening your abdominal muscles.
- Gently lower your hips back to the starting position, controlling the movement to maximize engagement of the core muscles.

The benefits of incorporating the Wall Jackknife into a senior's Wall Pilates routine are multifaceted. Firstly, it significantly strengthens the core muscles, which are pivotal for maintaining good posture, reducing back pain, and performing everyday activities with ease. Secondly, the controlled lifting and lowering motion enhances muscular endurance and promotes calorie burn, contributing to weight loss efforts. Additionally, the exercise improves flexibility in the hamstrings and lower back, areas where seniors often experience tightness and discomfort.

Moreover, the Wall Jackknife encourages the improvement of balance and coordination, as maintaining stability during the exercise requires a harmonious effort from various muscle groups. This enhanced balance is particularly beneficial for seniors, as it decreases the risk of falls and injuries, thereby promoting a more active and independent lifestyle.

While the Wall Jackknife is an advanced exercise, it's important for seniors to approach it with caution, starting slowly and gradually increasing the intensity as their strength and confidence grow. Consulting with a fitness professional or physical therapist before incorporating new exercises into their routine can provide personalized advice and modifications to ensure safety and effectiveness. Through consistent practice, the Wall Jackknife can become a valuable addition to a senior's weight loss and fitness regimen, offering both physical and mental health benefits that enrich their quality of life.

Wall Mountain Climbers

Wall Mountain Climbers in the context of Wall Pilates offer a dynamic, challenging exercise for seniors aiming to lose weight, while being mindful of the need for safety and adaptability. This variation of traditional mountain climbers uses the wall as a support, making it suitable for seniors who wish to engage in more advanced Pilates exercises without putting undue strain on their joints.

The exercise begins with the senior standing facing away from the wall, a few feet apart to allow for stability. They then place their hands on the floor, extending their legs behind them and resting their feet against the bottom of the wall. This starting position resembles a raised plank, with the body forming a straight line from head to heels, supported by the hands and feet.

- Start in a plank position: Position yourself so your hands are directly under your shoulders and your feet are up against the wall. Your body should form a straight line from your head to your heels.
- Engage your core: Before beginning the movement, tighten your abdominal muscles to stabilize your spine and pelvis.
- Begin the climbing motion: Gently bring one knee towards your chest, keeping the rest of your body stable. Then, return that foot to the starting position against the wall and switch legs, bringing the other knee towards your chest.
- Maintain a controlled pace: Continue alternating legs in a climbing motion. Focus on control and stability, rather than speed, to maximize engagement of your core muscles.
- Breathe consistently: Inhale and exhale smoothly throughout the exercise. Proper breathing not only aids in muscle activation but also increases the cardiovascular benefits of the exercise.

- Set a time or repetition goal: Start with shorter intervals or a lower number of repetitions, gradually increasing as your fitness level improves.

The benefits of Wall Mountain Climbers for seniors are multifaceted. Firstly, this exercise significantly enhances core strength, as the abdominal muscles are engaged to stabilize the body throughout the movement. Improved core strength contributes to better posture, reduced back pain, and enhanced overall mobility, making daily activities easier and more enjoyable.

Additionally, Wall Mountain Climbers are an excellent cardiovascular exercise, helping to increase heart rate and burn calories. This is particularly beneficial for weight loss, as consistent cardiovascular exercise is key to burning fat and improving metabolic health. The controlled pace and support from the wall ensure that the exercise remains safe for seniors, minimizing the risk of falls or injuries associated with balance issues.

Moreover, this exercise also strengthens the shoulders, arms, and legs, providing a comprehensive workout that enhances muscular endurance and flexibility. By incorporating Wall Mountain Climbers into their routine, seniors can enjoy a challenging yet safe way to elevate their fitness level and contribute to their weight loss goals.

The adaptability of Wall Mountain Climbers makes them a valuable addition to a senior's advanced Wall Pilates routine. For those new to the exercise, starting with a lower wall position or reducing the range of motion can help ease into the movement. As strength and confidence grow, the challenge can be increased, either by raising the feet higher on the wall or by incorporating longer intervals or more repetitions.

Incorporating Wall Mountain Climbers into a Wall Pilates routine for seniors not only aids in weight loss but also promotes a sense of achievement and progress. It exemplifies the principle that age should not be a barrier to engaging in challenging physical activities. By following the structured approach and recognizing the comprehensive benefits, seniors can safely enjoy the rewards of this advanced exercise, contributing to a healthier, more active lifestyle.

Wall Split

The Wall Split is an advanced exercise within the realm of Wall Pilates, especially designed for seniors aiming to lose weight and enhance their overall physical fitness. This exercise is notable for its ability to target and stretch the hamstrings, improve flexibility in the hips and legs, and strengthen the core muscles. While it may seem daunting at first, with patience and practice, it becomes an achievable milestone for those who have gradually built their foundation in Wall Pilates. Below are detailed instructions on how to perform the Wall Split, followed by its numerous benefits.

To perform the Wall Split, follow these steps:

- Begin by warming up your body with gentle stretches or a series of basic Wall Pilates exercises to prepare your muscles.
- Lie on your back on a mat, positioning yourself so that your buttocks are as close to a wall as possible. Your legs should be straight up against the wall, forming an L shape with your body.
- Slowly, start to open your legs into a split, letting them fall gently towards either side, maintaining a position where they are supported by the wall. Keep the movement controlled and stop at the point where you feel a comfortable stretch, not pain.

- Place your arms in a comfortable position, either by your sides or stretched out to the sides, palms facing up, to help maintain balance and open up the chest.
- Breathe deeply and hold the position for 1-3 minutes, depending on your comfort level. Focus on relaxing into the stretch with each exhale.
- To come out of the Wall Split, gently use your hands to support your legs as you bring them back together. Bend your knees towards your chest, roll to one side, and use your arms to help you sit up slowly.
- Finish with a few gentle stretches or movements to ensure your muscles are not shocked by the transition.

The benefits of incorporating the Wall Split into a senior's Wall Pilates routine are manifold. Primarily, this exercise offers an excellent way to improve lower body flexibility, which is crucial for maintaining a full range of motion, reducing the risk of falls, and performing daily activities with ease. Stretching the hamstrings, inner thighs, and hips can alleviate tightness and reduce discomfort, promoting better posture and mobility.

Moreover, the Wall Split encourages core engagement. As seniors work to maintain the split position against the wall, they must activate their abdominal muscles to stabilize their spine and pelvis. This not only enhances core strength but also supports overall body alignment and balance, key components in preventing injuries and managing weight.

For seniors focused on weight loss, integrating the Wall Split into their exercise regimen can contribute to a more holistic approach to fitness. While this particular exercise is more about flexibility and strength than cardiovascular endurance, it plays a crucial role in a well-rounded workout plan that supports weight management. By improving flexibility and core strength, seniors may find it easier to perform a wider variety of exercises, including those with a higher caloric burn.

Additionally, the Wall Split can offer therapeutic benefits. The act of stretching and focusing on deep, controlled breathing during the exercise can have a calming effect on the mind and body. This can reduce stress levels, which is beneficial for weight loss, as high stress is often linked to weight gain.

The Wall Split is an advanced Wall Pilates exercise that offers seniors a pathway to improved flexibility, core strength, and overall physical wellness. Its role in a weight loss journey, while indirect, is nonetheless important, as it supports the body's ability to engage in a broader range of physical activities safely and effectively. With regular practice, patience, and proper technique, the Wall Split can be a rewarding addition to a senior's fitness regimen.

Wall Stand

The Wall Stand, an advanced exercise in the realm of Wall Pilates, offers seniors a gateway to unlocking a plethora of benefits tailored to weight loss and overall body strengthening. This exercise, though advanced, can be approached with caution and consistency, making it a valuable addition to a senior's Pilates routine. Here, we delve into the intricacies of performing the Wall Stand, coupled with its benefits, ensuring a comprehensive understanding for those looking to elevate their fitness journey.

To begin the Wall Stand, it's crucial to ensure proper alignment and execution to maximize benefits while minimizing the risk of injury. The process involves:

- Start by standing with your back against the wall, feet hip-width apart, and positioned a few inches away from the wall.

- Engage your core muscles, pressing the small of your back into the wall to maintain spinal alignment.
- Slowly walk your feet away from the wall while simultaneously sliding your back down the wall, as if you are sitting in an invisible chair.
- Aim to lower yourself to a point where your thighs are parallel to the floor, ensuring your knees are aligned over your ankles, not extending past your toes.
- Press your shoulders and the back of your head lightly against the wall, maintaining a straight, elongated spine.
- Hold this position for a count of 10 to 30 seconds, depending on your comfort and ability, breathing deeply throughout.
- To return to the starting position, engage your thigh and core muscles, pushing through your heels to slide back up the wall.

Incorporating the Wall Stand into a senior's Pilates regimen brings forth several benefits pivotal for those aiming to lose weight and enhance their physical health. Firstly, this exercise significantly engages the core, including the abdominal muscles, promoting improved posture and balance. Such core activation is essential for daily movements and helps prevent falls, a common concern among seniors.

Moreover, the Wall Stand targets and tones the lower body muscles—the quadriceps, hamstrings, glutes, and calves. Strengthening these muscles not only contributes to a leaner physique but also boosts metabolism, aiding in more efficient weight loss. The resistance element of this exercise, primarily using one's body weight, is particularly effective for seniors seeking to increase muscle mass without the stress of free weights.

This exercise also enhances joint flexibility and mobility, particularly in the knees and hips, which is crucial for maintaining functional movement.

Regular practice of the Wall Stand can lead to improvements in tasks such as walking, climbing stairs, and bending, making it a practical choice for seniors looking to retain their independence.

Another noteworthy benefit is the improvement in cardiovascular health. Although the Wall Stand is primarily a strength-based exercise, maintaining the position increases heart rate, contributing to cardiovascular endurance. This is vital for heart health and plays a role in weight management.

The Wall Stand also teaches body awareness and control, essential components of physical fitness at any age. Learning to maintain the body in a controlled, stationary position helps seniors become more attuned to their body's capabilities and limits, fostering a safer exercise environment.

Lastly, the mental discipline required to hold the Wall Stand position can have positive implications beyond physical health, including stress reduction and enhanced mental focus. The concentration needed to perform this exercise effectively encourages a mindful approach to exercise, connecting the body and mind in the pursuit of health and wellness.

The Wall Stand, when performed correctly and consistently, is an excellent advanced Wall Pilates exercise for seniors aiming to lose weight and improve their overall physical condition. Its benefits extend from strengthening major muscle groups to enhancing mental well-being, making it a comprehensive exercise choice for seniors dedicated to leading a healthier lifestyle.

Wall Mermaid Stretch

The Wall Mermaid Stretch is a graceful, yet powerful component of advanced Wall Pilates exercises, particularly beneficial for seniors focusing on weight loss and overall flexibility. This exercise, inspired by the fluidity and strength of a mermaid's movement, utilizes the wall as a stabilizing tool to deepen the stretch and enhance postural alignment. It's an elegant blend of stretching and strengthening, targeting the sides of the body, including the obliques, latissimus dorsi, and intercostal muscles, while also engaging the core.

Instructions:

- Begin by sitting sideways next to the wall, with your legs folded to one side and your hips as close to the wall as possible. Ensure one hand is on the floor for support, while your side closest to the wall is prepared to lean against it.
- Inhale deeply, and on the exhale, gently place your closest hand to the wall above your head against the wall. The other hand remains on the floor for stability.
- Press the palm against the wall and slowly slide it up, allowing your torso to lean away from the wall, creating a deep side stretch. Your free hand slides on the floor away from the wall, maintaining balance.
- Hold the position where a comfortable stretch is felt along the side body. Ensure not to overextend, and keep the sit bones grounded.
- Maintain the stretch for 15-30 seconds, focusing on deep, steady breaths that help deepen the stretch with each exhale.
- To release, gently slide the wall hand down, returning to the starting position.
- Repeat on the opposite side to ensure balanced stretching.

Benefits:

1. Improved Flexibility: This stretch deeply works the side muscles, promoting increased flexibility in the torso, hips, and shoulders, which can enhance the range of motion and reduce stiffness.

2. Enhanced Core Strength: By engaging the core throughout the stretch, seniors can improve their abdominal and lower back strength, contributing to better posture and balance.

3. Stress Reduction: The focused, deep breathing associated with this exercise aids in stress reduction and promotes relaxation, important for overall wellness and weight loss efforts.

4. Increased Circulation: The stretching motion helps boost circulation to the muscles being worked, facilitating oxygen and nutrient delivery, which is vital for muscle recovery and health.

5. Posture Improvement: Regularly performing the Wall Mermaid Stretch helps correct postural imbalances by lengthening tight muscles and strengthening underused ones, contributing to a more upright, confident posture.

Incorporating the Wall Mermaid Stretch into a Wall Pilates routine offers seniors a multifaceted exercise that not only aids in their weight loss journey by engaging and stretching the body in a gentle, yet effective way but also enhances their daily functional movements by improving flexibility and reducing muscle tension. It's a testament to the adaptability and benefits of Wall Pilates for seniors, proving that age should not be a barrier to achieving fitness and wellness goals.

Chapter 7: Special Focus Routines

Routine for Improving Balance

Improving balance is an important part of staying healthy and independent as we age, and Wall Pilates provides a unique, supportive technique for seniors to improve their stability while also losing weight. This unique practice combines Pilates concepts with the safety of a wall to provide a safe and effective approach for seniors to strengthen their core, improve their balance, and gradually work toward their weight reduction objectives.

The sequence begins with the Wall Roll Down, a fundamental exercise that elongates the spine and engages the core muscles, which are essential for balance. Participants stand with their backs to the wall and feet hip-distance apart. They progressively glide down the wall, vertebra by vertebra, until the head, shoulders, and upper back emerge from the wall, pausing to feel the core engagement before slowly rolling back up. This exercise warms up the body and prepares the muscles for the tasks ahead.

Next, the Wall Squat strengthens the legs and core, increasing stability. Seniors drop down into a squat posture with their backs on the wall, making sure their knees do not extend past their toes, before pressing back up. This action not only improves leg strength, which is essential for balance, but it also encourages core engagement, which is required to maintain an upright posture.

The Side Wall Lifts work on the obliques and enhance lateral balance, allowing seniors to manage shifts in their center of gravity. Seniors stand sideways to the wall, one hand supporting them, and lift their leg closest to the wall sideways before lowering it with control. This exercise tests their balance and strengthens the side muscles of the belly and legs.

The Wall Plank focuses on the entire core, which is necessary for proper balance. Seniors face the wall, hands at shoulder height, and step back until their body forms a straight line from head to heels, activating their abdominal muscles. Holding this stance strengthens the core and shoulders, increasing overall stability.

Toe Taps are included in the program to improve coordination and ankle stability, both of which are important for balance. Seniors face the wall for support and lift one foot off the ground, softly tapping the toes down in front of them, then to the side, and lastly behind them, repeating the pattern many times before moving on to the other foot. This workout improves not just balance, but also coordination and flexibility in the lower body.

The heel raises are executed with the back against the wall. Seniors lift their heels off the ground, onto their toes, and then gently descend back down. This strengthens the calf muscles and increases proprioception, which is necessary for balance.

Finally, the practice closes with the Wall Push-Up, which, while predominantly an upper-body exercise, needs core engagement and stability, bringing together the strength and balance training from the whole routine. Seniors face the wall, hands slightly wider than shoulder width, bend their elbows to bring their bodies closer to the wall, then push back to their starting position. This exercise guarantees that the upper body is also involved in the balance-improving process.

Seniors who incorporate this Wall Pilates practice into their weekly plan will progressively improve their balance, strengthen their core, and contribute to their weight loss objectives. Aside from the physical advantages, the program provides mental and emotional boosts, providing seniors a sense of accomplishment and confidence in their movements, lowering the chance of falling, and encouraging a more active, independent living. Through persistent practice, seniors can experience the combined benefits of enhanced balance and getting closer to their weight control targets, generating a holistic feeling of well-being.

Routine for Enhancing Flexibility

Wall Pilates, with its unique combination of support and resistance, provides an excellent avenue for seniors looking to improve their flexibility while losing weight. Flexibility is an important component of total fitness, particularly as we age, as it allows for more mobility, lower chance of injury, and a higher quality of life. A regimen developed expressly to improve flexibility can considerably help with these aims, making daily tasks simpler and more pleasurable.

This specific practice starts with an emphasis on warming up the body, which is an important step in preparing the muscles and joints for stretching and preventing tension. Standing arm circles and wall-assisted walking in place are two basic yet powerful warm-up exercises. These motions stimulate blood flow and gently mobilize the shoulders and hips, laying the groundwork for the flexibility exercises that follow.

The routine's core consists of a sequence of wall-assisted stretches that target specific muscle groups such as the hamstrings, back, shoulders, and hips. The Wall Hamstring Stretch is a basic exercise in which seniors lay their heel on a low stool near the wall and slowly lean forward, allowing the wall to maintain their balance. This stretch may be held for 15-30 seconds and performed on both sides. It is very useful for relaxing tight hamstrings, which are frequent among seniors.

Following the hamstring stretch, the practice progresses to the Wall Angel exercise, which is a great action for expanding the chest and shoulders. Standing with their backs against the wall, seniors lift their arms in a "W" formation and gently glide them up and down, replicating the action of snow angels. This exercise not only improves shoulder flexibility but also prevents the forward slouch that typically occurs with aging.

The Cat-Cow Stretch, modified for the wall, is another essential component of the practice. Seniors can place their hands on the wall at waist height, take a step back, and alternate between arching their back toward the wall (cow) and rounding it away (cat). This action increases spinal flexibility and can help relieve lower back stiffness, allowing for a more fluid range of motion.

The Wall Pigeon stance is a safe version of the conventional yoga stance that helps with hip flexibility. Seniors can utilize a chair against the wall for support by gently placing one leg on the chair in a bent posture and extending the other behind, utilizing the wall for balance. This stretch focuses on the hip flexors and glutes, which are essential for mobility but typically grow stiff with age.

The last stretches are followed by a concentration on deep, regulated breathing, stressing the relationship between breath and movement. This not only helps to deepen each stretch, but also promotes relaxation and stress relief. The last steps of the program might include a basic Wall Lean, in which elders lean into the wall with their arms extended, take deep breaths, and allow gravity to gently stretch their entire body.

Incorporating this program into a weekly plan, possibly two to three times per week, can progressively improve flexibility, helping a senior achieve their weight reduction objectives by allowing for more rigorous exercise with less discomfort. It's critical to approach each exercise with care and to listen to the body's signals, changing the stretches to meet personal limitations and guarantee safety.

This Routine for Increasing Flexibility within the Wall Pilates framework is intended to be accessible, effective, and pleasant for older citizens. It not only helps them lose weight but also improves their overall quality of life, demonstrating that flexibility and mobility can be improved at any age.

Routine for Strengthening the Core

In the world of Wall Pilates for seniors looking to reduce weight and improve their overall health, a practice centered on core development is essential. The core, as the body's center of power, has an important function in stabilizing the entire body, improving posture, and lowering the chance of injury, making it a key area for seniors to address. This customized practice includes a sequence of exercises that gently but efficiently target the muscles of the belly, back, and pelvis, increasing strength and stability in these regions.

The workout starts with the Wall Roll Down, which is a great exercise for stimulating the deep core muscles. Standing with the back against the wall, seniors can carefully roll down vertebra by vertebra, lowering the chin to the chest and slightly bending the knees to keep the lower back in touch with the wall. This action not only warms up the body, but also promotes a connection with the core muscles, preparing them for the next activity.

The Wall Plank then uses an isometric hold to test the core while reducing pressure on the lower back. Participants face away from the wall and lay their hands on the ground, stretching their feet back until their heels push on the wall. The pose is kept for many breaths, keeping a straight line from head to heels and working the core muscles the entire time. For those who want a less strenuous alternative, place the forearms on the ground when performing this exercise.

Moving on to the Wall Bridge, seniors lie on their backs, feet flat on the wall and knees bent. They exercise the glutes and hamstrings as well as the core by forcing their feet against the wall and raising their hips to the ceiling. This exercise strengthens the lower back and abdominal muscles while also improving pelvic stability, which is essential for balance and movement.

The Standing Leg Lift tests the core's stability and strength. Standing parallel to the wall, seniors can use one hand to support the opposite leg while lifting it to the side, maintaining the pelvis firm and the core engaged. This exercise not only works the obliques, but it also improves coordination and balance, which are important components of a healthy and active lifestyle for seniors.

Using the Wall Scissors adds a dramatic challenge to the routine. Seniors lie on their backs with their legs elevated against the wall, alternately moving one foot down to the floor and back up, imitating a scissor action. This action necessitates strong core engagement to maintain stability, especially as the legs move independently of one another.

To achieve a complete core exercise, the program includes Wall Mountain Climbers, which have been modified for seniors by placing hands on a wall rather on the floor. This variant puts less pressure on the wrists and shoulders while yet activating the entire core as seniors alternately pull their knees to their chest in a controlled manner.

After the intense core training, the exercise concludes with a gentle Wall Push-Away stretch that decompresses the spine. Standing arm's length from the wall, seniors press against it with their hands, rounding the back and tucking the chin, feeling a stretch in the back and sides of their bodies. This not only cools the body but also maintains flexibility and strength.

This Wall Pilates practice for core strength is specifically created for seniors, providing a balanced approach to increasing core strength, improving balance, and contributing to a better weight reduction path. Seniors who incorporate these exercises into their regular fitness routine may get the many benefits of a strong, stable core, such as a lower chance of falling, improved posture, and a higher capacity to do daily activities with ease and confidence.

Routine for Lower Back Pain Relief

Lower back discomfort is a frequent condition among seniors, sometimes impeding an active lifestyle and weight control. Wall Pilates, which focuses on core strength, flexibility, and posture, is a mild yet effective way to relieve lower back pain. Incorporating Wall Pilates into your daily routine not only helps you lose weight, but it also improves your general spinal health, which is important for seniors looking to improve their quality of life.

The program for lower back pain recovery with Wall Pilates begins with an emphasis on core activation. The abdominals, back, and pelvic muscles all play an important part in supporting the spine. Strengthening these regions can greatly reduce tension on the lower back, hence relieving discomfort. The Wall Roll Down is an excellent exercise in which elders stand with their backs to the wall, feet hip-width apart, and slightly away from the wall. They then slowly slide down the wall, vertebra by vertebra, tucking the chin into the chest and bending the knees to keep the core engaged throughout the action. This exercise enhances spinal flexibility and core activation, both of which are necessary for addressing lower back discomfort.

Another important part of the practice is the Wall Pelvic Tilt. This exercise focuses on pelvic mobility, which can help relieve lower-back stress. Seniors would press their lower back toward the wall, straining their abdominal muscles and thrusting the pelvis slightly forward, before relaxing. Repeating this action strengthens the lower abdominal muscles and extends the lower back, reducing pain.

Incorporating leg strengthening exercises into your program can also help support your lower back. The Wall Sit, for example, not only strengthens the thighs and buttocks, but it also promotes appropriate posture and alignment, which are essential for decreasing lower back pain. Seniors may strengthen their lower bodies by sliding down the wall into a sitting posture with their knees at a 90-degree angle and holding it.

Flexibility exercises, such as the Wall Stretch, are also useful. Seniors can stretch their back and hamstring muscles by standing arm's length away from the wall, reaching up to placing their palms on the wall, and leaning gently forward. This stretch not only relieves lower back tightness but also develops hamstring flexibility, which is significant because tight hamstrings can cause lower back discomfort.

Breathing skills, which are central to Pilates, are stressed throughout the practice. Proper breathing helps to oxygenate the muscles, relieves tension, and promotes relaxation. Focusing on deep, controlled breaths during exercises can increase their efficiency and give a relaxing effect, lowering the stress that frequently aggravates lower back discomfort.

It is critical for seniors to listen to their body and tailor the intensity of their activities to their comfort levels. The practice should begin with a few repetitions and progress as strength and flexibility improve. Consistency is crucial; following this program on a regular basis can result in considerable reductions in lower back discomfort, making it simpler for seniors to engage in everyday activities and continue their weight loss journey.

Finally, combining this Wall Pilates program with a healthy diet and adequate water is critical for weight control and general wellness. By addressing lower back discomfort with specific exercises, seniors can have more mobility, less pain, and an enhanced capacity to pursue their weight reduction objectives, demonstrating the overall advantages of Wall Pilates in encouraging a healthier, more active lifestyle for elders.

Chapter 8: Integrating Wall Pilates into Your Daily Life

Designing Your Weekly Wall Pilates Schedule

Integrating Wall Pilates into the everyday lives of seniors who want to lose weight requires considerable preparation and attention to develop a long-term and successful weekly regimen. This approach begins with a comprehension of older persons' particular physical demands and time limits, as well as the fact that a well-structured program may result in considerable gains in health, mobility, and weight management over time.

A well-designed weekly Wall Pilates routine for seniors should begin with the concept of progressive growth. For people new to Pilates or returning to physical exercise after a period of idleness, two to three sessions per week are recommended. These sessions, which last between 20 and 30 minutes, allow the body to adjust to new motions without producing undue stress or weariness. As strength, flexibility, and endurance improve, the frequency and duration of sessions can be increased, with the objective of achieving three to four sessions per week lasting up to 45 minutes each.

Diversity in routine is essential for meeting seniors' holistic health and fitness goals. Each session should include a range of exercises for different muscular groups, such as the core, legs, arms, and back. This not only eliminates boredom, but also offers a comprehensive approach to body strengthening and toning. Exercises that promote balance and flexibility, such as the Wall Plank or Standing Leg Lifts, can also help to reduce falls and improve general mobility.

Recovery time is critical for seniors who participate in Wall Pilates. Rest days in between workouts are vital for muscle recovery and injury prevention. On these days, simple exercises like walking or moderate stretching might assist preserve mobility without overworking the body. Listening to one's body and modifying training intensity or taking extra rest days as needed is essential for maintaining a good and healthy attitude to weight reduction and fitness.

Wall Pilates workouts should be timed consistently to match the individual's natural energy levels throughout the day. Some people find morning workouts stimulating and a terrific way to start the day, but others prefer afternoon or early evening activities when they are more attentive and nimbler. Consistency in scheduling not only helps to develop a habit, but also guarantees that Pilates becomes an integrated part of everyday life.

It is impossible to stress the importance of having a warm-up and cool-down phase in each practice. Begin with mild stretches and basic motions to prepare the body for more strenuous activity, lowering the chance of injury. Ending each session with a cool-down phase that includes stretches and relaxation methods promotes muscle healing and flexibility, hence increasing the overall efficacy of the Wall Pilates program.

Finally, including mindfulness and breathing methods into the weekly routine increases the mental and emotional advantages of Wall Pilates. Focusing on breath control and mindfulness during exercises can enhance attention, reduce stress, and boost body awareness, enhancing the entire Wall Pilates experience for seniors. This comprehensive approach not only helps with weight reduction, but it also promotes overall well-being and healthy living.

A weekly Wall Pilates routine for seniors comprises a mix of scheduled exercise, rest, and mindfulness techniques. Seniors may experience the full advantages of Wall Pilates by adapting the routine to their own requirements and preferences, accomplishing their weight reduction objectives while also enhancing their physical and mental health.

Tracking Your Progress

Integrating Wall Pilates into the everyday lives of seniors, particularly those looking to reduce weight, entails more than simply regular exercise; it also requires a rigorous approach to measuring progress. This rigorous tracking is critical not just for assessing physical gains and weight reduction, but also for increasing motivation and changing the training schedule for best outcomes. Tracking success in Wall Pilates may be a difficult task that includes both qualitative and quantitative changes over time.

The essence of progress monitoring is to develop unambiguous, quantitative success markers. For seniors who practice Wall Pilates, these signs might range from the number of sessions completed each week to gains in specific exercises, such as higher repetitions or the capacity to do more advanced motions with greater comfort. Furthermore, documenting weight reduction with frequent weigh-ins or body measurements gives actual proof of bodily changes, which encourages and reinforces the efficacy of their efforts.

Beyond numerical statistics, qualitative factors of advancement are vital. Seniors might keep a personal diary to track physical and emotional changes. This might include observations of improved energy, better sleep quality, or a general sense of well-being. Such qualitative indicators are frequently the first evidence of improvement, even before obvious weight reduction or bodily changes, making them an effective motivator.

The use of technology allows for a more efficient way to tracking development. Several applications and digital platforms are available to help you log exercises, track weight reduction, and even get reminders for scheduled Pilates sessions. These digital tools might help seniors focus on their workouts rather than the administrative difficulties of tracking their success. Furthermore, some apps allow users to see progress over time using graphs and data, providing a clear image of how far they have come.

Setting frequent review points is another important part of progress tracking. Seniors may make educated decisions about altering their Pilates regimen by scheduling regular review and assessment sessions, whether weekly or monthly. These assessments can indicate patterns, such as which exercises produce the best results or when times of day are most energetic, allowing for a more tailored and successful training schedule.

Accountability relationships or joining a Wall Pilates group designed particularly for elders can also help measure progress. Sharing objectives and progress with peers fosters a sense of community and support, which promotes consistency and devotion. Group settings may also provide possibilities for friendly competition or shared milestone celebrations, which can motivate individuals to keep working hard.

Reflecting on progress is a strong reminder of the journey and the successes made. Looking back and recognizing how far they've come may be quite satisfying for seniors. It's important to appreciate the improvements in strength, flexibility, and general health along the journey, rather than merely achieving the ultimate objective of weight loss. Celebrating these accomplishments, whether they be learning a new Pilates exercise or observing a good shift in body composition, promotes a positive mentality and emphasizes the significance of living an active lifestyle.

To summarize, measuring success in Wall Pilates for seniors who want to lose weight is a thorough process that includes both the physical and mental components of their trip. Seniors who meticulously assess their progress can stay motivated, change their habits for better outcomes, and eventually live a healthier, happier lifetime. Tracking not only provides a road map to success, but it also acts as a transformation diary, charting the path to better health and vitality.

Staying Motivated and Overcoming Plateaus

Integrating Wall Pilates into the everyday lives of seniors, particularly those seeking to reduce weight, is a path fraught with possible highs and unavoidable plateaus. Maintaining motivation during these ebbs and flows is critical for long-term performance and general well-being. Any exercise plan, including Wall Pilates, has periods of quick success as well as times when changes appear to stagnate. Understanding and managing these stages with grace and drive can make all the difference in meeting one's health objectives.

Setting clear, attainable goals, as previously noted, can help motivate people, but it also demands a deeper, internal desire. This motivation is frequently motivated by a recognition of Wall Pilates' greater advantages beyond weight reduction, such as increased flexibility, better posture, and improved mental clarity. When progress on the scale slows, non-scale successes are critical for keeping excitement and dedication to one's practice. Seniors can stay motivated by reflecting on these changes on a frequent basis and contemplating their influence on everyday living, such as being able to complete daily activities more easily or enjoying longer walks with less weariness.

Overcoming plateaus in weight reduction and fitness necessitates a diversified strategy. A plateau might suggest that the body has acclimated to the present level of activity and need a fresh challenge to go forward. For seniors who practice Wall Pilates, this might entail adding more complex movements to their regimen or increasing the frequency or duration of their sessions. To avoid harm, make these changes gradually and pay close attention to the body's indications.

Variety is not just the spice of life; it is also an essential component in maintaining motivation and breaking past plateaus. Changing patterns, attempting new Wall Pilates movements, or incorporating activities like walking or swimming may rekindle interest and challenge the body in novel ways. This variety helps to work different muscle areas and can restart progress in weight reduction and fitness.

Another important part of remaining motivated is the power of community and support. Seniors can tremendously benefit from participating in Wall Pilates groups or courses, as well as discussing their experience with others who share their aims. This sense of community creates a network of support and accountability, making it easier to stay motivated even when progress appears to stagnate. Sharing experiences, struggles, and accomplishments with people who understand the path may offer a major emotional lift and serve as a reminder that one is not alone in overcoming these obstacles.

Setting and praising modest, intermediate accomplishments is an effective method for staying motivated. Rather of focusing primarily on a long-term weight loss goal, creating smaller, more feasible goals can create a sense of success and motivation. Celebrating these milestones, such as buying a new book, taking a soothing bath, or going on a social event, may reinforce positive behaviors and develop a sense of accomplishment over time.

Finally, it is critical to cultivate a patient and compassionate perspective. Progress in weight reduction and fitness, particularly among seniors, is not usually linear. There will be weeks when everything falls into place naturally, and others when keeping a schedule feels difficult. Recognizing that these swings are a normal part of the process allows for a gentler, more forgiving attitude to personal development. It is critical to recognize the work put in, even if the results are not immediately obvious.

Finally, including Wall Pilates into your everyday life as a senior looking to lose weight is a journey full of hurdles and victories. Staying motivated during the highs and overcoming the inevitable plateaus takes a combination of strategic modifications, community support, celebration of minor accomplishments, and a healthy dose of patience and self-care. By adopting these tactics, seniors can not only achieve their weight reduction and exercise objectives, but also improve their entire quality of life.

Chapter 9: Nutrition and Diet for Weight Loss

Basics of Nutrition for Seniors

Understanding the fundamentals of nutrition is critical for seniors, particularly those commencing on a weight loss journey with techniques such as Wall Pilates. As the body ages, its nutritional requirements change, making it critical for seniors to modify their diets to maintain optimal health, support active lives, and aid in weight reduction. Wall Pilates, recognized for its gentle yet effective method to increasing strength and flexibility, complements a well-structured food plan designed to meet the specific needs of older persons.

A balanced diet for seniors focuses on nutrient-dense foods that give high nutritional value without consuming too many calories, which is necessary for weight management and maintaining the energy requirements of a Pilates practice. Incorporating a variety of fruits and vegetables is essential since they are high in vitamins, minerals, and fiber yet low in calories. These nutrients promote muscular health, which is especially important for seniors who do Wall Pilates, as the exercises frequently rely on core strength and stability. Furthermore, the fiber in these meals assists digestion and helps maintain a healthy weight by giving you a sense of fullness, which reduces the probability of overeating.

Protein consumption is another important aspect of senior nutrition, particularly for individuals who engage in exercise such as Wall Pilates. Adequate protein promotes muscle repair and development, which is essential for seniors seeking to enhance their physical fitness and reduce weight. Lean protein foods such as poultry, fish, beans, and lentils can help maintain muscle mass without adding too much fat to the diet. Seniors should distribute their protein intake throughout the day to promote continual muscle synthesis and recuperation following Pilates exercises.

Healthy fats should not be disregarded in a senior's diet, especially if they are trying to lose weight or practice Pilates. Fish, nuts, and seeds include omega-3 fatty acids, which are essential for joint health, cognitive function, and inflammation reduction. These benefits are especially important for seniors who practice Wall Pilates, which focuses on joint mobility and flexibility. Incorporating healthy fats may help give a consistent energy supply, improving endurance throughout Pilates sessions.

Seniors' general well-being and weight loss attempts rely heavily on proper hydration. As one matures, the sense of thirst decreases, increasing the danger of dehydration. Drinking plenty of water boosts metabolism, promotes digestion, and allows muscles to perform properly throughout Pilates workouts. Seniors should drink water throughout the day and avoid sugary beverages, which can add unneeded calories to their diet.

Micronutrients, such as vitamins D and B12, calcium, and iron, are essential for seniors, especially those who want to reduce weight using Wall Pilates. These nutrients promote bone health, energy, and general physical function. Seniors may need to pay extra attention to certain micronutrients since absorption diminishes with age. To ensure that these nutritional needs are satisfied, consider including fortified meals or visiting a healthcare practitioner about supplements.

Finally, adjusting portion sizes and eating behaviors can have a substantial influence on weight reduction attempts in seniors who do Wall Pilates. Eating smaller, more frequent meals can help balance blood sugar levels, control appetite, and give steady energy throughout the day. This strategy also meets the energy demands of seniors who do Pilates on a daily basis, providing a consistent supply of nutrients to sustain their activity levels.

Seniors may build a strong synergy by combining Wall Pilates with a well-rounded, healthy diet that promotes weight loss, increases muscular strength and flexibility, and improves overall health. Recognizing and adjusting to the aging body's unique dietary demands is critical in this journey, allowing seniors to enjoy active, satisfying lives.

Diet Tips for Enhancing Pilates Weight Loss

When seniors begin a Wall Pilates practice to lose weight, using certain food suggestions can greatly improve their results. Pilates, particularly for seniors, such as Wall Pilates, focuses on core strength, flexibility, and total muscular tone. A well-balanced and healthy diet is necessary to supplement these physical advantages. This combination of targeted exercise and mindful eating can speed weight loss and generate a deeper sense of well-being.

First and foremost, water is essential in any weight loss effort. Drinking enough water boosts metabolism, aids in the effective burning of calories, and guarantees that the body operates properly throughout Pilates workouts. Seniors should consume water throughout the day, especially before and after their Wall Pilates workouts, to keep hydrated and energized. Incorporating herbal teas can give hydration while also providing antioxidant advantages.

Protein consumption is critical for muscle repair and growth, especially in Pilates, which often tests and improves muscular strength. Seniors should consume lean protein sources such chicken, fish, tofu, lentils, and low-fat dairy products. These proteins help with post-workout recovery and muscle mass maintenance, both of which are necessary for a healthy metabolism.

Fruits and vegetables are essential in a diet designed to improve Pilates weight reduction. These food categories are high in vitamins, minerals, and fiber, yet low in calories. They fill you up without adding unnecessary calories, making weight management easier. Seniors should aim to fill half of their plate with a colorful array of fruits and vegetables at each meal to ensure they obtain a full range of nutrients.

Whole grains are another key ingredient. Brown rice, quinoa, whole wheat pasta, and oats are good sources of slow-release energy. This consistent supply of energy is essential for seniors to get through their Pilates exercises and throughout the day, avoiding blood sugar spikes that can lead to cravings and overeating.

Healthy fats shouldn't be disregarded. Avocados, almonds, seeds, and olive oil are good sources of satiety, promote heart health, and lower inflammation. These facts are especially advantageous for seniors because they provide the calories required for energy without the negative consequences associated with saturated and trans fats.

Meal time can also have an impact on Pilates' ability to help people lose weight. Eating smaller, more balanced meals and snacks throughout the day might help keep the metabolism going and give a continuous supply of energy for exercise and everyday activities. This technique can help to reduce overeating at meals while still ensuring that the body gets the nutrition it requires to work and recover properly.

Finally, mindful eating is a practice that is consistent with the concepts of Pilates. Paying attention to hunger cues, eating slowly, and enjoying food might help with digestion and overall meal pleasure. It promotes a healthy connection with food and helps seniors avoid overeating by making them more aware of their bodies' true demands.

Seniors who practice Wall Pilates for weight reduction might get better results if they follow these diet guidelines. A balanced, healthy diet helps to meet the physical demands of Pilates, nourishes the body effectively, and supplements the workout's advantages for a more holistic approach to health and wellness. This combination of conscious activity and food can lead to a healthier, more vibrant existence in our golden years.

Easy and Nutritious Recipes

Incorporating Wall Pilates into a senior's weight reduction regimen is a step toward a healthy living. However, combining physical activity with a nutritious diet can dramatically increase the advantages of exercise. Easy and healthful foods are especially important for seniors beginning on this journey. These recipes not only help them achieve their fitness objectives, but also respond to their changing nutritional demands, ensuring that their meals benefit their entire health and well-being.

The balance of macronutrients—proteins, carbs, and fats—is essential for any healthful weight reduction diet plan. High-quality protein sources, such as lean meats, fish, lentils, and dairy, are essential for muscle repair and maintenance, especially for seniors who practice Wall Pilates. Including a reasonable quantity of complex carbs in meals, such as whole grains, vegetables, and fruits, offers the energy needed for workouts and everyday tasks. Healthy fats, such as avocados, nuts, seeds, and olive oil, are essential for joint health and cognitive function.

One simple meal that exemplifies this balance is quinoa and black bean salad. Quinoa is a complete protein and a good source of complex carbs, while black beans provide fiber and extra protein. A variety of bright vegetables, such as bell peppers and spinach, provide additional vitamins, minerals, and antioxidants. Tossed with an olive oil and lemon juice dressing, this salad is not only nutritional but also heart-healthy and anti-inflammatory, making it an excellent dinner for seniors.

Smoothies are another great alternative for seniors, since they provide a simple and digestible approach to get a range of nutrients. A smoothie containing spinach, banana, blueberries, Greek yogurt, and a tablespoon of flaxseed contains a high concentration of protein, omega-3 fatty acids, calcium, fiber, and antioxidants. This combination promotes muscular health, bone density, and digestive health while being pleasant to the palette and quick to prepare.

Baked salmon with roasted sweet potatoes and green beans is a hearty lunch with a good balance of lean protein, complex carbs, and fiber. Salmon has a lot of omega-3 fatty acids, which are good for your heart and help reduce inflammation. Sweet potatoes are a low glycemic index carbohydrate source high in vitamins A and C, while green beans offer crunch and fiber. This meal promotes fullness and nutrient density, making it not only enjoyable but also beneficial to a healthy weight reduction journey.

Soup is another adaptable and senior-friendly option, with lentil soup being a favorite. Lentils are a great source of plant-based protein and fiber, which help you feel full and ease digestion. Adding a variety of veggies, such as carrots, tomatoes, and kale, boosts the soup's nutritious content, delivering critical vitamins and minerals without adding too many calories. Seasoned with spices such as turmeric and cumin, it has anti-inflammatory properties as well as a warming taste.

Finally, a simple grilled chicken and veggie wrap may be a nutritious and easy supper for seniors. This meal has a whole grain wrap, lean grilled chicken breast, and a variety of fresh veggies including lettuce, cucumber, and bell peppers. A spread of hummus or avocado adds healthy fats and taste, making it a filling meal that promotes weight loss and muscle maintenance.

Incorporating these simple and healthy meals into a senior's diet will greatly help them achieve their weight reduction and health objectives when combined with Wall Pilates. These meals not only supply the nutrition their bodies require to fuel and recuperate from exercises, but also respond to their changing dietary demands, allowing them to enjoy great, nutritious meals without the burden of intricate preparations. Focusing on nutrient-dense, balanced meals, seniors may improve their overall wellbeing, making their journey with Wall Pilates both successful and pleasurable.

Conclusion

To conclude the investigation of Wall Pilates as a transforming tool for seniors looking to lose weight, it's important to consider the journey's importance and the larger influence of such a practice on one's life. Wall Pilates, with its gentle yet effective approach, is more than simply a technique to lose weight; it is a comprehensive journey to better health, increased mobility, and a stronger connection between mind and body. This type of exercise, designed expressly for the requirements and limits of seniors, emphasizes the notion that age should never be an impediment to reaching one's health and fitness objectives.

The Wall Pilates journey for weight reduction in seniors highlights the significance of setting realistic objectives, knowing one's body's individual demands, and gradually incorporating this kind of exercise into everyday life. The wall provides safety, stability, and support in these activities, allowing seniors to engage in physical activity without fear of damage, making it an excellent solution for individuals worried about balance and stability. As seniors develop in their practice, they notice not only physical improvements, such as weight reduction and enhanced flexibility, but also mental and emotional advantages, such as higher self-esteem and a sense of success.

Wall Pilates' adaptable nature allows for training customization and adjustment, guaranteeing that each individual may work at their own speed and alter their program to meet their changing fitness levels. This flexibility is essential for sustaining a steady practice that challenges and benefits the body while avoiding strain or discomfort. Furthermore, because Wall Pilates requires no equipment, it can be done practically anyplace, encouraging people to include it into their daily routines.

The communal component cannot be ignored. Seniors who participate in Wall Pilates frequently find themselves part of a supportive community, whether through group sessions, online forums, or casual encounters. This sense of belonging can boost motivation and dedication to one's health objectives by offering not just physical but also social and emotional support.

Reflecting on my weight reduction experience with Wall Pilates, it is evident that the advantages go far beyond the physical. This technique promotes a mindful approach to exercise, focusing on the process rather than the outcome. It promotes a connection to one's body that many people haven't felt in years, allowing for a gentle yet powerful form of self-expression and self-care.

To summarize, Wall Pilates stands out as an excellent type of exercise for seniors wanting to lose weight, providing a multidimensional approach that targets physical, mental, and emotional wellness. It demonstrates that with the correct mentality, adequate goals, and a dedication to one's well-being, age can truly become a number. The Wall Pilates journey for seniors is about more than simply reducing weight; it's about having a fuller, more vibrant experience of life, distinguished by mobility, strength, and a strong feeling of personal accomplishment.

28 Days Program

Day	Focus Area	Exercise	Repetitions / Duration
1	Full Body	Wall Squats, Wall Push-ups	2 sets of 10-12 reps
2	Core & Balance	Standing Knee Lifts, Wall Plank	2 sets of 10-12 reps
3	Lower Body	Wall Sit, Heel Raises	2 sets of 10-12 reps
4	Rest or Gentle Stretching	Gentle Wall Stretching	5-10 minutes
5	Upper Body & Core	Wall Push-ups, Standing Oblique Crunches	2 sets of 10-12 reps
6	Flexibility & Balance	Wall-assisted Leg Stretches, Toe Touches	2 sets of 10-12 reps

7	Rest or Gentle Stretching	Gentle Wall Stretching	5-10 minutes
8	Full Body	Wall Push-ups, Wall Squats, Standing Knee Lifts	2 sets of 10-12 reps
9	Core & Lower Body	Wall Plank, Wall Sit	2 sets of 10-12 reps
10	Upper Body & Flexibility	Wall Push-ups, Wall-assisted Chest Stretch	2 sets of 10-12 reps
11	Rest or Gentle Stretching	Gentle Wall Stretching	5-10 minutes
12	Balance & Core	Standing Oblique Crunches, Wall Plank	2 sets of 10-12 reps
13	Lower Body	Wall Sit, Heel Raises	2 sets of 10-12 reps

14	Rest or Gentle Stretching	Gentle Wall Stretching	5-10 minutes
15	Full Body	Wall Squats, Wall Push-ups, Standing Knee Lifts	2 sets of 10-12 reps
16	Core & Flexibility	Wall Plank, Wall-assisted Leg Stretches	2 sets of 10-12 reps
17	Upper & Lower Body	Wall Push-ups, Wall Sit	2 sets of 10-12 reps
18	Rest or Gentle Stretching	Gentle Wall Stretching	5-10 minutes
19	Balance & Core	Standing Knee Lifts, Standing Oblique Crunches	2 sets of 10-12 reps
20	Full Body	Wall Squats, Wall Push-ups, Wall Plank	2 sets of 10-12 reps

Day	Focus	Exercises	Duration/Reps
21	Rest or Gentle Stretching	Gentle Wall Stretching	5-10 minutes
22	Core & Lower Body	Wall Sit, Heel Raises, Wall Plank	2 sets of 10-12 reps
23	Flexibility & Balance	Wall-assisted Leg Stretches, Toe Touches	2 sets of 10-12 reps
24	Rest or Gentle Stretching	Gentle Wall Stretching	5-10 minutes
25	Full Body	Wall Push-ups, Wall Squats, Standing Knee Lifts	2 sets of 10-12 reps
26	Core & Upper Body	Wall Plank, Wall Push-ups	2 sets of 10-12 reps
27	Lower Body & Flexibility	Wall Sit, Wall-assisted Leg Stretches	2 sets of 10-12 reps

| 28 | Rest or Gentle Stretching | Gentle Wall Stretching | 5-10 minutes |

15 DAYS WORKOUT JOURNAL TRACKER

DAILY WORKOUT TRACKER

DATE

DAILY MOTIVATION

TODAY'S GOALS

WEATHER

EXECERCISE TYPE

AMOUNT OF WATER

TOTAL :

JOGGING

TOTAL MINUTES

TOTAL STEPS

TODAY'S WORKOUT PLAN

TIME	WORKOUT TYPE

WORKOUT TO GET DONE TODAY

EXERCISE COMPLETED

HEALTHY DIET TRACKER

BREAKFAST	LUNCH
DINNER	SNACKS

NOTES

WORKOUT FOR

DAILY WORKOUT TRACKER

DATE

DAILY MOTIVATION

TODAY'S GOALS

WEATHER

EXECERCISE TYPE

AMOUNT OF WATER

TOTAL :

JOGGING

TOTAL MINUTES

TOTAL STEPS

TODAY'S WORKOUT PLAN

TIME	WORKOUT TYPE

WORKOUT TO GET DONE TODAY

EXERCISE COMPLETED

HEALTHY DIET TRACKER

BREAKFAST	LUNCH
DINNER	SNACKS

NOTES

WORKOUT FOR

DAILY WORKOUT TRACKER

DATE

DAILY MOTIVATION

TODAY'S GOALS

WEATHER

EXECERCISE TYPE

AMOUNT OF WATER

TOTAL :

JOGGING

TOTAL MINUTES

TOTAL STEPS

TODAY'S WORKOUT PLAN

TIME	WORKOUT TYPE

WORKOUT TO GET DONE TODAY

EXERCISE COMPLETED

HEALTHY DIET TRACKER

BREAKFAST | LUNCH

DINNER | SNACKS

NOTES

WORKOUT FOR

DAILY WORKOUT TRACKER

DATE

DAILY MOTIVATION

WEATHER

TODAY'S GOALS

EXECERCISE TYPE

AMOUNT OF WATER

TOTAL :

JOGGING

TOTAL MINUTES

TOTAL STEPS

TODAY'S WORKOUT PLAN

TIME	WORKOUT TYPE

WORKOUT TO GET DONE TODAY

EXERCISE COMPLETED

HEALTHY DIET TRACKER

BREAKFAST	LUNCH
DINNER	SNACKS

NOTES

WORKOUT FOR

DAILY WORKOUT TRACKER

DATE

DAILY MOTIVATION

TODAY'S GOALS

WEATHER

EXECERCISE TYPE

AMOUNT OF WATER

TOTAL :

JOGGING

TOTAL MINUTES

TOTAL STEPS

TODAY'S WORKOUT PLAN

TIME	WORKOUT TYPE

WORKOUT TO GET DONE TODAY

EXERCISE COMPLETED

HEALTHY DIET TRACKER

BREAKFAST	LUNCH
DINNER	SNACKS

NOTES

WORKOUT FOR

DAILY WORKOUT TRACKER

DATE

DAILY MOTIVATION

TODAY'S GOALS

WEATHER

EXECERCISE TYPE

AMOUNT OF WATER

TOTAL :

JOGGING

TOTAL MINUTES

TOTAL STEPS

TODAY'S WORKOUT PLAN

TIME	WORKOUT TYPE

WORKOUT TO GET DONE TODAY

EXERCISE COMPLETED

HEALTHY DIET TRACKER

BREAKFAST	LUNCH
DINNER	SNACKS

NOTES

WORKOUT FOR

DAILY WORKOUT TRACKER

DATE

DAILY MOTIVATION

WEATHER

TODAY'S GOALS

EXECERCISE TYPE

AMOUNT OF WATER

TOTAL :

TODAY'S WORKOUT PLAN

TIME	WORKOUT TYPE

WORKOUT TO GET DONE TODAY

JOGGING

TOTAL MINUTES

TOTAL STEPS

EXERCISE COMPLETED

HEALTHY DIET TRACKER

BREAKFAST	LUNCH
DINNER	SNACKS

NOTES

WORKOUT FOR

DAILY WORKOUT TRACKER

DATE

DAILY MOTIVATION

TODAY'S GOALS

WEATHER

EXECERCISE TYPE

AMOUNT OF WATER

TOTAL :

JOGGING

TOTAL MINUTES

TOTAL STEPS

TODAY'S WORKOUT PLAN

TIME	WORKOUT TYPE

WORKOUT TO GET DONE TODAY

EXERCISE COMPLETED

HEALTHY DIET TRACKER

BREAKFAST	LUNCH
DINNER	SNACKS

NOTES

WORKOUT FOR

DAILY WORKOUT TRACKER

DATE

DAILY MOTIVATION

TODAY'S GOALS

WEATHER

EXECERCISE TYPE

AMOUNT OF WATER

TOTAL :

JOGGING

TOTAL MINUTES

TOTAL STEPS

TODAY'S WORKOUT PLAN

TIME	WORKOUT TYPE

WORKOUT TO GET DONE TODAY

EXERCISE COMPLETED

HEALTHY DIET TRACKER

BREAKFAST	LUNCH
DINNER	SNACKS

NOTES

WORKOUT FOR

DAILY WORKOUT TRACKER

DATE

DAILY MOTIVATION

TODAY´S GOALS

WEATHER

EXECERCISE TYPE

AMOUNT OF WATER

TOTAL :

JOGGING

TOTAL MINUTES

TOTAL STEPS

TODAY´S WORKOUT PLAN

TIME	WORKOUT TYPE

WORKOUT TO GET DONE TODAY

EXERCISE COMPLETED

HEALTHY DIET TRACKER

BREAKFAST	LUNCH
DINNER	SNACKS

NOTES

WORKOUT FOR

DAILY WORKOUT TRACKER

DATE

DAILY MOTIVATION

TODAY'S GOALS

WEATHER

EXECERCISE TYPE

AMOUNT OF WATER

TOTAL :

JOGGING

TOTAL MINUTES

TOTAL STEPS

TODAY'S WORKOUT PLAN

TIME	WORKOUT TYPE

WORKOUT TO GET DONE TODAY

EXERCISE COMPLETED

HEALTHY DIET TRACKER

BREAKFAST	LUNCH
DINNER	SNACKS

NOTES

WORKOUT FOR

DAILY WORKOUT TRACKER

DATE

DAILY MOTIVATION

TODAY'S GOALS

WEATHER

EXECERCISE TYPE

AMOUNT OF WATER

TOTAL :

JOGGING

TOTAL MINUTES

TOTAL STEPS

TODAY'S WORKOUT PLAN

TIME	WORKOUT TYPE

WORKOUT TO GET DONE TODAY

EXERCISE COMPLETED

HEALTHY DIET TRACKER

BREAKFAST	LUNCH
DINNER	SNACKS

NOTES

WORKOUT FOR

DAILY WORKOUT TRACKER

DATE

DAILY MOTIVATION

TODAY'S GOALS

WEATHER

EXECERCISE TYPE

AMOUNT OF WATER

TOTAL :

TODAY'S WORKOUT PLAN

TIME	WORKOUT TYPE

WORKOUT TO GET DONE TODAY

JOGGING

TOTAL MINUTES

TOTAL STEPS

EXERCISE COMPLETED

HEALTHY DIET TRACKER

BREAKFAST	LUNCH
DINNER	SNACKS

NOTES

WORKOUT FOR

DAILY WORKOUT TRACKER

DATE

DAILY MOTIVATION

TODAY'S GOALS

WEATHER

EXECERCISE TYPE

AMOUNT OF WATER

TOTAL :

JOGGING

TOTAL MINUTES

TOTAL STEPS

TODAY'S WORKOUT PLAN

TIME	WORKOUT TYPE

WORKOUT TO GET DONE TODAY

EXERCISE COMPLETED

HEALTHY DIET TRACKER

BREAKFAST	LUNCH
DINNER	SNACKS

NOTES

WORKOUT FOR

DAILY WORKOUT TRACKER

DATE

DAILY MOTIVATION

TODAY'S GOALS

WEATHER

EXECERCISE TYPE

AMOUNT OF WATER

TOTAL :

TODAY'S WORKOUT PLAN

TIME	WORKOUT TYPE

WORKOUT TO GET DONE TODAY

JOGGING

TOTAL MINUTES

TOTAL STEPS

EXERCISE COMPLETED

HEALTHY DIET TRACKER

BREAKFAST	LUNCH
DINNER	SNACKS

NOTES

WORKOUT FOR

www.ingramcontent.com/pod-product-compliance
Lightning Source LLC
Chambersburg PA
CBHW050823260726
48660CB00004B/1571